100 Questions & Answers About Asthma

Second Edition

Claudia S. Plottel, MD

Clinical Associate Professor
Department of Medicine
Division of Pulmonary and Critical Care Medicine
NYU School of Medicine
NYU–Langone Medical Center
New York, NY

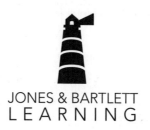

JONES & BARTLETT
L E A R N I N G

616,238
PLO

World Headquarters

Jones & Bartlett Learning
40 Tall Pine Drive
Sudbury, MA 01776
978-443-5000
info@jblearning.com
www.jblearning.com

Jones & Bartlett Learning
Canada
6339 Ormindale Way
Mississauga, Ontario L5V 1J2
Canada

Jones & Bartlett Learning
International
Barb House, Barb Mews
London W6 7PA
United Kingdom

Jones & Bartlett Learning books and products are available through most bookstores and online booksellers. To contact Jones & Bartlett Learning directly, call 800-832-0034, fax 978-443-8000, or visit our website, www.jblearning.com.

Substantial discounts on bulk quantities of Jones & Bartlett Learning publications are available to corporations, professional associations, and other qualified organizations. For details and specific discount information, contact the special sales department at Jones & Bartlett Learning via the above contact information or send an email to specialsales@jblearning.com.

The author, editor, and publisher have made every effort to provide accurate information. However, they are not responsible for errors, omissions, or for any outcomes related to the use of the contents of this book and take no responsibility for the use of the products and procedures described. Treatments and side effects described in this book may not be applicable to all people; likewise, some people may require a dose or experience a side effect that is not described herein. Drugs and medical devices are discussed that may have limited availability controlled by the Food and Drug Administration (FDA) for use only in a research study or clinical trial. Research, clinical practice, and government regulations often change the accepted standard in this field. When consideration is being given to use of any drug in the clinical setting, the healthcare provider or reader is responsible for determining FDA status of the drug, reading the package insert, and reviewing prescribing information for the most up-to-date recommendations on dose, precautions, and contraindications, and determining the appropriate usage for the product. This is especially important in the case of drugs that are new or seldom used.

Production Credits
Executive Publisher: Christopher Davis
Editorial Assistant: Sara Cameron
Production Director: Amy Rose
Associate Production Editor: Laura Almozara
Associate Marketing Manager: Marion Kerr
Manufacturing and Inventory Control Supervisor: Amy Bacus
Composition: Glyph International
Printing and Binding: Malloy, Inc.
Cover Design: Colleen Lamy/Carolyn Downer
Cover Image: Top left photo: © Levent Konuk/ShutterStock, Inc.; Top right photo: © Wendy Kaveney Photography/ShutterStock, Inc.; Middle photo: © Denis Mironov/ShutterStock, Inc.; Bottom photo: © Photos.com
Cover Printing: Malloy, Inc.

Library of Congress Cataloging-in-Publication Data
Plottel, Claudia S.
  100 questions & answers about asthma / Claudia Plottel. — 2nd ed.
      p. cm.
  Includes bibliographical references and index.
  ISBN-13: 978-0-7637-8091-3 (alk. paper)
  ISBN-10: 0-7637-8091-X (alk. paper)
  1. Asthma—Popular works. 2. Asthma—Miscellanea. I. Title. II. Title:
One hundred questions and answers about asthma.
  RC591.P574 2011
  616.2'38—dc22
                                                        2010011422

6048

Printed in the United States of America
14 13 12 11 10   10 9 8 7 6 5 4 3 2 1

Contents

Preface   vii

Abbreviations   xi

Part One: Asthma: Facts, Theories, and Controversies   1

Questions 1–12 provide the latest information about asthma, including:
- What is asthma?
- Why is asthma so common?
- How do human lungs work?
- What causes asthma?
- What is the relationship between allergy and asthma?
- What is the contemporary view of asthma and how does it differ from traditional views?

Part Two: Asthma: Symptoms and Diagnosis   33

Questions 13–31 describe the symptoms of asthma and present common methods of diagnosis, such as:
- What are the symptoms of asthma?
- What is an exacerbation of asthma?
- Does wheezing mean that I have asthma?
- Are there medical conditions that can mimic asthma or make it more severe?
- How is the diagnosis of asthma established?
- What are pulmonary function tests (PFTs), spirometry, and peak expiratory flow (PEF) measurements?

Part Three: Asthma: Classification and Variants   67

Questions 32–40 introduce the NAEPP's approach to asthma care and review atypical forms of asthma, including:
- What is the National Asthma Education and Prevention Program (NAEPP)?
- What is cough-variant asthma?
- What is the asthmatic triad?
- What is occupational asthma?
- What is an asthma action plan?
- Why should I take asthma medicine if I feel fine?

Part Four: Asthma: Treatment Plans, Goals, and Strategies   95

Questions **41–53** detail key components of asthma care that underlie effective treatment, such as:

- What are asthma triggers?
- What are the goals of asthma treatment?
- What makes a doctor an asthma specialist and how can I find out if my physician is a specialist in asthma care?
- Do I need to consult a physician who specializes in asthma?
- My asthma is active; how do I know whether I should go to the nearest hospital emergency room?

Part Five: Asthma: Inhaled Medications and Advances   127

Questions **54–71** focus on the different medications used to treat asthma, with an emphasis on inhaled formulations:

- What medications are useful in treating asthma?
- Will I need to take asthma medicine forever?
- Why are so many asthma medicines in inhaler form?
- What is the correct way to use my dry-powder inhaler (DPI)?
- What is the correct way to use my metered-dose inhaler (MDI)?
- What are corticosteroids and how do they work in asthma?

Part Six: Asthma: A Healthy Lifestyle   187

Questions **72–83** highlight day-to-day living with asthma, including:

- What are the newest approaches to the treatment of asthma?
- Can acupuncture or herbal remedies help my asthma? Will alternative or complementary medicine treatments be good for my asthma?
- My asthma seems to worsen each month around the time of my period. Is that possible?
- Is obesity related to asthma?
- What sports can persons with asthma participate in?
- Is asthma mostly a psychological disease?

Part Seven: Special Topic: Asthma and Pregnancy   235

Questions **84–88** answer the most common questions of women with asthma who become pregnant, such as:

- Will pregnancy make my asthma worse?
- Can I do anything special during my pregnancy to help protect my unborn child from developing asthma in the future?
- Are asthma medications harmful to the unborn child?
- Will I be able to breastfeed my baby if I am taking medicine for my asthma?

Part Eight: Special Topic: Asthma in Children   245

Questions 89–100 respond to everyday parental concerns when a child has asthma, for instance:

- Can I catch asthma from my child who has asthma?
- Do milk products cause increased mucus in persons who have asthma, especially children?
- Should I take my four-year-old to a physician who specializes in asthma? Can the primary care pediatrician diagnose and treat her asthma?
- Will my child outgrow his asthma?
- How can I help my son's school staff cope with his asthma and know how to handle an emergency?
- Our 10-year-old daughter who has asthma wants to go to sleep-away camp next summer. Should she attend a regular camp or a camp for children with asthma?

Appendix 1   267

Appendix 2   273

Glossary   283

Index   305

Contents

"The good of a book lies in its being read."

The Name of the Rose (1981) Umberto Eco (1932–)

The very first question that comes to mind once you've glanced at the cover of *100 Questions & Answers About Asthma, Second Edition,* might well be: "Why read a book on the topic of asthma?" One answer invokes the ongoing asthma epidemic. Asthma affects more than 22 million Americans, including 7.3% of the adult population and 6.7 million children. The numbers reflect the fact that we all know at least one person who has been diagnosed with asthma. Perhaps, like many of my own friends and relatives, you want to ask questions about the asthma care and advice you have received from your doctor. You want to know more, understand asthma better, and learn about contemporary developments and advances.

The next question you will most likely ask me is: "Why have you now written a second edition of the book—is anything new or different?" Much has transpired in the world of asthma in the six years since the first edition went to press. I chose to keep the overall organization of the book unchanged, and this second edition updates all but a handful of the questions covered in the first edition. I have added information about the latest scientific approaches to asthma care and research, elucidated the newest guidelines and treatment recommendations of the National Asthma Education and Prevention Program, and included comprehensive facts about the medicines used to treat asthma. The focus remains, as always, on healthy living with asthma, so you will again find answers to your questions about exercise and diet. As in the first edition, there are special sections dedicated to the most common questions about asthma in pregnancy and asthma in children, as well as a glossary and a listing of print and Internet asthma resources for your reference.

The last question you'll ask me is more personal: "Why do you write books on asthma?" I am a lung specialist, board certified in internal medicine as well as in pulmonary medicine, with a specific interest in asthma care, particularly in adults. In the more than 25 years since I graduated from medical school, the medical community's understanding of asthma has increased tremendously, our views on effective treatment have changed a great deal, and highly effective medicines have been developed and brought to market. Successful asthma treatment, however, includes more than prescriptions for medication. It requires an accurate exchange of information, which goes hand-in-hand with effective communication. The 100 questions I selected for inclusion in this book are real questions that have been put to me over the years in the hospital, clinic, and office.

100 Questions & Answers About Asthma, Second Edition, provides scientific, accurate, and timely information that reflects both the medical profession's current understanding of asthma and my personal experience as an asthma specialist. The question-and-answer format allows you to flip through the book and read ahead to those topics that most interest you, in any order that you choose. The questions are also ordered in such a manner that you can read them in sequence. Gemma Goode, who has carried a diagnosis of asthma for most of her life, kindly and graciously agreed to offer a patient's perspective on successful living with asthma. Her point of view is complemented by Kerrin Robinson's perceptive insights into caring for her young son with asthma. You will find their comments in italics throughout the book.

I wish to acknowledge Christopher Davis, Executive Publisher for Medicine at Jones & Bartlett Learning, who has been steadfast in his support for *100 Questions & Answers About Asthma, Second Edition.* I am grateful to Laura Almozara, Associate Production Editor at Jones & Bartlett Learning, for her all-around expertise and to Janet Kiefer for her copyediting skills. Special heartfelt thanks to Larry, Charles, and Elisabeth Stam, enthusiastic readers and staunch supporters!

Preparing the updated and revised *100 Questions & Answers About Asthma, Second Edition,* has, just as the first edition did, challenged me to think about how best to communicate medical information and facts, and how to explain "the doctor's side" of asthma. I have greatly enjoyed researching and writing the book you now have before you. My hope is that you will learn as much from reading *100 Questions & Answers About Asthma, Second Edition*, as I did from writing it.

Claudia S. Plottel, MD

Preface

The following is a list of commonly used abbreviations in asthma care that appear throughout the text.

DPI   dry-powder inhaler
FEV_1 forced expiratory volume in 1 second
FVC   forced vital capacity
HFA   hydrofluoroalkane
ICS   inhaled corticosteroid
LABA   long-acting β_2 (beta$_2$) agonist
LTRA   leukotriene receptor antagonist
MDI   metered-dose inhaler
OCS   oral corticosteroid
SABA   short-acting β_2 (beta$_2$) agonist
VHC   valved holding chamber

PART ONE

Asthma: Facts, Theories, and Controversies

What is asthma?

Why is asthma so common?

How do human lungs work?

What causes asthma?

What is the relationship between allergy and asthma?

What is the contemporary view of asthma
and how does it differ from traditional views?

More . . .

Asthma

A chronic respiratory condition characterized by breathing symptoms of varying intensity and frequency.

Wheeze

The abnormal sound produced when air travels in and out through a narrowed breathing passage or breathing tube. The narrowing in asthma can be due to a constriction of the breathing tube or accumulated mucus, or both.

A major goal of asthma treatment is directed at symptom prevention as well as at symptom control.

Mucus

A mixture composed of water, salt, and proteins produced by specialized cells in the nose, sinuses, and lung passages. Mucus plays a defensive role and helps to protect from infection.

"C'est une ennuyeuse maladie que de conserver sa santé par un trop grand régime."

"It is a wearisome illness to preserve one's health by too strict a regimen."

—La Rochefoucauld (1613–1680), *Maximes*

1. What is asthma?

Asthma is a very common, highly treatable lung condition. Millions of individuals worldwide, children and adults, carry a diagnosis of asthma. Asthma's symptoms relate to breathing and to the respiratory system. Symptoms of asthma vary in frequency and in intensity and may include cough, wheeze, increased mucus production, uncomfortable breathing, and shortness of breath. Asthma severity not only varies from person to person, but can also fluctuate in a given person over time. A major goal of asthma treatment is directed at symptom prevention as well as at symptom control. Some people with mild asthma experience infrequent symptoms. Others, whose asthma is more persistent, at the other end of the asthma severity spectrum, may require several daily lung medications taken regularly to control their disease, normalize their lung functioning, and attain a symptom-free state.

Physicians who specialize in asthma care firmly believe that even the most severely affected asthma sufferers can be treated successfully. Modern asthma management and contemporary therapies allow persons diagnosed with asthma to lead full, active lives. Successful asthma treatment requires an understanding of the disease in general as well as how it manifests itself in a particular person, combined with attentive medical care and the forging of a cooperative partnership between patient and physician (Table 1).

Table 1   Components of Contemporary Asthma Treatment

- Medications tailored to asthma severity and degree of control
- Environmental control measures
- Immunizations (including against influenza)
- Identification and treatment of any co-existing medical conditions
- Patient, family, and caregiver education
- Self-management strategies and guidelines
- Regular aerobic exercise
- Forging of a true therapeutic alliance between patient and healthcare provider

2. How many Americans have asthma?

Asthma is a very common lung disease. It has been described in all ethnic groups and in all ages, from childhood into the golden years. The U.S. Centers for Disease Control and Prevention's (CDC's) National Center for Health Statistics reports that asthma currently affects more than 22.2 million Americans or 7.9% of the population, including over 6.7 million children younger than 18 years of age (Table 2). Another way of looking at the information is that 7.3% of American adults currently have asthma, as do 9.3% of all young persons aged 15 years or younger (Table 3). Asthma is the most common chronic disease of childhood. It is also the primary cause of school absences due to a chronic condition. Young people aged 5–17 years with asthma miss more than 12.8 million school days annually in the United States. Asthma is responsible for interference with adults' daily activities as well, given that over 10 million work days are lost annually to poorly controlled asthma.

The cost of asthma is significant both for individuals and for our society as a whole. Experts refer to the burden of asthma. The CDC estimates that in 2006,

Asthma is the most common chronic disease of childhood.

Chronic

Longstanding, lingering, or expected to last indefinitely; as opposed to acute.

Table 2   Asthma in the United States

- Approximately 22.2 million Americans currently have asthma, including 6.7 million children aged 18 years or less—the numbers correspond to 7.3% of adults and 9.3% of children.
- Asthma is the most common chronic disease of childhood.
- In 2006, asthma accounted for 10.6 million visits to office-based physicians, 1.3 million visits to hospital clinics, and 1.8 million visits to hospital emergency departments.
- Asthma is responsible for 12.8 million missed school days and 10 million missed days of work each year.
- There were 3613 reported deaths in the United States in 2006 directly due to asthma. Asthma is a contributing factor in nearly 7000 additional deaths.
- Asthma-related health costs amount to $19.7 billion annually in the United States.

Source: Adapted from data obtained via the Centers for Disease Control and Prevention, including the brochure: Breathing Easier; accessed via: http://www.cdc.gov/asthma/pdfs/breathing_easier_brochure.pdf

Table 3   The Centers for Disease Control and Prevention's (CDC) Data on Asthma Prevalence Rates By Age, Gender, and Race in the United States— As Assessed in 2006

U.S. Population	% with Asthma
Children	9.3%
Adults	7.3%
Male	7.0%
Female	8.6%
White	7.9%
Black	9.2%
Hispanic	6.4%

The prevalence of asthma is an assessment of the total number of persons in the United States that have been diagnosed with asthma as counted in 2006, no matter how long the disease has been present. Prevalence data include both "new" and "old" cases and indicate how many persons are affected with asthma at a given point in time.

Source: National Health Interview Survey, National Center for Health Statistics, Centers for Disease Control and Prevention

asthma accounted for 10.6 million visits to office-based physicians, 1.3 million visits to hospital clinics, and 1.8 million visits to hospital emergency departments. The rate of emergency department visits for asthma was higher in children than in adults, and the highest rate of asthma requiring emergency department care was for children 4 years of age and younger. Hospitalizations for asthma appear to be decreasing over recent years, and presently approximate close to half a million yearly, with higher rates of hospitalization among children than among adults. The highest rate of hospitalization for treatment of asthma, similar to the rate of emergency room utilization is for children aged 4 and younger.

Experts are interested in reducing the burden of asthma illness and the rates of hospitalization in the United States as in all other countries. The fact that the hospitalization rates for asthma in the United States have been decreasing may reflect the beneficial effects of the introduction of newer asthma therapies, including medications such as those referred to as "controller" or "maintenance" medicines, reviewed later in the text. This book will help you learn about asthma and good management practices, and it will present strategies that may assist you in better understanding your condition. Knowing that asthma is so common serves as a reminder that you are far from alone. Properly treated asthma allows for a full and rewarding lifestyle, and that fact, along with the fact that millions of American have been diagnosed with asthma, explains why you will see persons with asthma achieve just about everything, everywhere! I have met athletes with asthma, teachers with asthma, actors with asthma, and lawyers and doctors with asthma. As one patient of mine confided with a grin, "Doc, if I can brush and floss my teeth twice a day every day of my life, what's the big deal with taking a few more minutes to inhale medicine that keeps me healthy?"

3. Is it true that asthma is on the upswing?

Yes, asthma has increased steadily in the United States through the 1980s and 1990s, as in other Westernized countries. There are more persons diagnosed with asthma now than ever before in the United States. The prevalence of asthma—that is the total number of cases of asthma in a population at any given point in time— continues to increase worldwide (Table 4). It may also be true that allergic conditions are on the increase. The reason why asthma is increasing in the United States and in other industrialized nations is unclear. A far-reaching international effort to understand the scope of increasing asthma (and allergy) in young people led in 1991 to the formation of the ambitious and ongoing International Study of Asthma and Allergies in Childhood, known as ISAAC, and accessible on the Internet at http://isaac.auckland.ac.nz/. ISAAC describes itself as "the largest worldwide collaborative research program ever undertaken involving more than 100 countries and 2 million children." Findings that have emerged from the ISAAC study include the observation that

There are more persons diagnosed with asthma now than ever before in the United States.

Table 4   Prevalence of Asthma: International Patterns

- Asthma is increasing worldwide.
- Asthma is generally more common in Western countries as compared to developing countries.
- Asthma is more prevalent in English-speaking countries.
- Asthma prevalence is increasing in developing countries as they become more urbanized and more "Westernized."
- There appears to be an accompanying increase in allergic diseases as well.

Source: Adapted from: Beasley R, Crane J, Lai CK, Pearce N. Prevalence and etiology of asthma. *J Allergy Clin Immunol.* 2000;105:S466–472.

English-speaking countries demonstrate the highest prevalence rates for asthma and that Latin American countries also have elevated asthma rates.

Of great concern to physicians are certain urban neighborhoods, such as the South Bronx and East Harlem in New York City, where rates of asthma hospitalization and asthma deaths are among the highest in the nation, and where nearly 20% of children have been diagnosed with asthma. When looking at "the big picture" however, U.S. data collected from 1980 to 1996 reveal, as mentioned previously, an increase in asthma prevalence. Since 1995, there have also been increases in national rates of office, clinic, and emergency room visits for asthma. Those increases developed in parallel with a decrease in the rates of hospitalization for asthma and of deaths from asthma. Experts believe that the increase in the number of outpatient visits is the result of better and more effective asthma treatment in the setting of increasing numbers of persons diagnosed with the disease. The recorded drop in hospital admissions for asthma and the reductions in the death rate are also consistent with improved asthma care overall—an encouraging public health statistic!

Gemma's comment:

Is asthma more common in urban than rural areas? Environmental factors are very important in the city, but many of the triggers that plague urban environments may also be found in rural areas, such as volatile organic compounds (found in varnishes, aerosol sprays, household disinfectants, and similar products), peeling paint, mold, decaying wood in older buildings, not to mention the heavy smoke from those romantic wood fires that vacationers love to build when they go to the country. My own childhood was spent in a small, midwestern town with no significant heavy industry or other causes of environmental pollution, yet it was marked for me by an annual parade of seasonal allergies, colds, and a perpetual, wheezing croup.

4. Why is asthma so common?

Asthma is very common, affecting approximately one of every ten Americans at some point in their life, according to 2001 data from the CDC's National Health Interview Survey. It is not clear why asthma has become such a prevalent, chronic condition. One theory holds that physicians have become more adept at diagnosing asthma correctly so that the more precise identification and more accurate counting of persons with asthma has led to a perceived increase in diagnosed cases of asthma. Unfortunately, the opposite is true—the diagnosis of asthma is too often overlooked, particularly in older age groups and in adolescents, especially in teenage girls. The fact is that asthma has truly become more common. A more likely theory implicates various environmental factors. Smoking, for example, became socially acceptable for women after World War II. Infants of mothers who smoke are at risk for the development of wheezing and asthma in childhood. Increasing air pollutants and small particles found in urban or industrial areas may also play an important role. More information about the possible causes of asthma is presented in Question 8. From the perspective of an asthma specialist, the greater awareness of the importance of air quality in general and the enactment of laws banning smoking in all indoor public places, such as in New York City, in particular are a crucial step toward improving air quality for all.

5. Asthma is a disease of children, isn't it?

Asthma affects people of all ages, as mentioned in Question 2, and a diagnosis of asthma can be made in a child as young as 2 years of age. Asthma is the most common chronic disease of childhood. Asthma is not, however, a disease limited to children. It is a myth that asthma is only a disease of childhood, and that all children with asthma will outgrow their asthma with time as they grow into adulthood, as explained in Question 95. Many persons newly diagnosed with asthma are adults. Although some adults with asthma may have experienced asthma as a child, others develop the condition the first time as an adult. Asthma can thus develop at any age.

6. How do human lungs work?

The lungs are the major component of the respiratory system (Figures 1A and 1B). A good way to understand the workings of the lungs is to consider their structure, or anatomy (Figure 1A). The human respiratory system begins at the nose and includes the nasal passages, which direct air to the back of the throat and into the windpipe, or trachea. The trachea sits below the voice box (larynx), and can be felt in the front of your neck as it descends behind the breastbone (sternum) into the upper chest. The trachea ends and divides into two branches: the right mainstem bronchus and the left mainstem bronchus. The right mainstem bronchus leads air to and from the right lung, and the left mainstem bronchus leads air to and from the left lung.

The area where the trachea divides into the right and left mainstem bronchi is called the carina. After the split, the right and left mainstem bronchi leading to each lung subdivide further into smaller and smaller tubelike passages, via the branching tracheobronchial tree. As the bronchi continue to subdivide into successively narrower and narrower bronchi, they ultimately end in the tiniest subdivision, the bronchiole. Each bronchiole leads to the lung air sacs, the alveoli.

Trachea

The scientific name for the windpipe. The trachea leads air from the back of the nose and mouth into the lungs.

Carina

The split where the lungs' trachea divides into two branches— the right mainstem bronchus and the left mainstem bronchus, which lead air to the right lung and left lung, respectively.

Bronchus (plural bronchi)

A breathing passage or tube. The trachea splits at the level of the carina into the right and left mainstem bronchi.

Bronchiole

The fine, tapered, thin-walled breathing passages that branch and extend from the bronchus, and end in the alveolar air sacs.

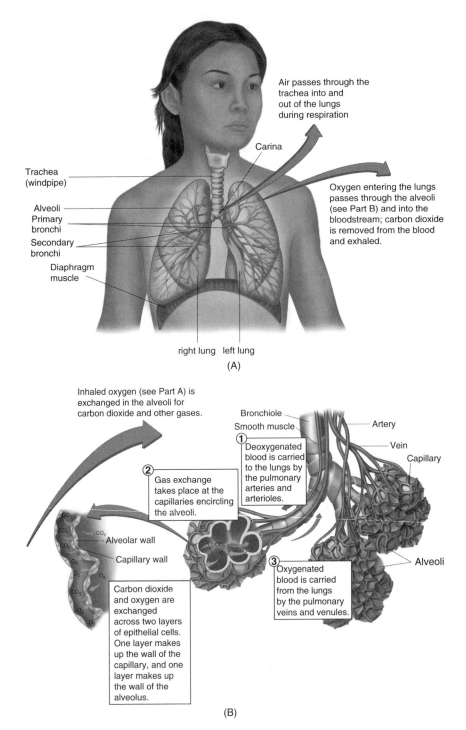

Figure 1   The Lungs and Breathing: (A) Anatomy and (B) Respiration.

The alveoli are highly specialized lung structures. They are the gas-exchanging lung units. They ensure that fresh, oxygen-rich (O_2) inhaled air enters the body at the same time that oxygen-poor, carbon dioxide-rich (CO_2) air exits (Figure 1B). Oxygen (O_2) is required for life; oxygen deprivation is rapidly fatal. As inhaled oxygen is provided to the body's organs via the lungs, "used" air—composed mostly of carbon dioxide (CO_2)—is excreted by exhalation. Carbon dioxide is produced by the body's metabolism and is considered a "waste product." Abnormal accumulation of carbon dioxide in the body and the bloodstream is detrimental to health and is responsible for certain forms of respiratory failure.

The process that is responsible for the body's oxygen uptake and its carbon dioxide removal (or excretion) is called respiration. Respiration is the primary, crucial function of the lungs and of the respiratory system. Physicians occasionally refer to respiration as "gas exchange." The exchanged gases are oxygen (O_2) and carbon dioxide (CO_2). Exchange means that CO_2 gas is given up by the body and replaced by a fresh supply of O_2. The exchange takes place in the deepest lung, at the level of the alveoli. Oxygen and carbon dioxide exchange takes place along a specialized zone where each air sac (alveolus) is in intimate contact with fine, minute blood vessels called capillaries. The capillary bed completely encircles the alveoli along the alveolar–capillary membrane. Because of the structure of the alveolar-capillary membrane, the inhaled oxygen (O_2) easily passes from the alveolus into the capillary blood that then sends it to our organs. Similarly, the body's CO_2 is carried through the bloodstream into the blood supply of the alveolar–capillary membrane where it is given up to the alveolus, and from there, exhaled by our lungs with each breath. A normal resting adult breathes

Oxygen (O_2)

An odorless, colorless gas necessary for life. The air we breathe is comprised of 21% oxygen.

Carbon dioxide (CO_2)

An odorless, colorless gas produced as a waste by-product by the body's metabolism.

Gas exchange

The process by which O_2 and CO_2 enter and leave the body, via the lungs' alveolar capillary membrane.

Capillary

A tiny, thin-walled blood vessel. The word is derived from capillus, the Latin word for hair.

Alveolar-capillary membrane

The alveolar-capillary membrane is the interface between the alveolar surface and the blood circulation.

approximately 12–18 times a minute, children about 20 times a minute, and babies and infants even more frequently. That number, the number of breaths a person breathes in 1 minute, is termed the *respiratory rate*. We should be unaware of our breathing in health, as respiration should be automatic, effortless, and of course, painless. Increases in the respiratory rate, sometimes perceived as a kind of breathless sensation, can represent a normal process as during exercise or sports and allows for increased oxygen delivery to the body. A respiratory rate increase can also indicate the onset of a medical concern; it may in particular be a sign of increasing asthma symptomatology. That is why measurement of respiratory rate, along with pulse (or heart rate), blood pressure, and temperature measurements are collectively referred to as vital signs in medical terminology!

We should be unaware of our breathing in health, as respiration should be automatic, effortless, and of course, painless.

Respiratory rate

The number of breaths one takes in a minute.

7. Do lungs continue to develop after birth?

Yes, our lungs continue to grow and develop after we are born. In particular, the specialized gas-exchanging lung units called alveoli, where oxygen is exchanged for carbon dioxide, develop postnatally. The majority of the lung alveoli—nearly 85%—are in fact formed after birth, during the first 3 years of life. The blood supply within the capillary network matures in parallel with alveolar development from birth to 3 years of age. Mucus cells that line the air passages also develop after birth.

Alveolus (plural: alveoli)

An alveolus is a lung's air sac. Oxygen is exchanged for carbon dioxide in the lung alveoli. A healthy adult human lung contains approximately 300 million alveoli.

Postnatally

After birth. Human lungs continue to grow and develop postnatally, into infancy.

Because the majority of alveoli develop postnatally, the first 3 years of life after birth can be viewed as an especially vulnerable period. Experts believe that poorly controlled asthma in childhood and adolescence may be responsible for reduced lung capacity and lessened lung function throughout life. In addition to controlling childhood asthma, it is crucial that babies and children be raised in smoke-free homes to maximize normal lung maturation.

After the age of 3, the lungs are formed, but not fully grown. As our bodies develop through adolescence to adulthood, so too, do our lungs. Adolescence represents a second vulnerable window. Recent scientific studies indicate that teenagers who smoke are left with lung function that is less than that of healthy nonsmoking teens. The finding of stunted lung function development in adolescent smokers is especially notable in girls.

8. What causes asthma?

Asthma is believed to result from a complex interplay between a person's genes and various environmental factors at a specific time in his or her life. It can thus be viewed as the result of interactions that occur between internal (genetic) elements and external (environmental) exposures. Environmental factors that have been studied include viruses such as RSV (respiratory syncytial virus), cockroaches, cigarette smoke, exhaust, farm animals, medications (including acetaminophen), pesticides, pets, and wood smoke. The data are intriguing and raise further questions that continue to stimulate research both into genetic and environmental features. Recent attention has, for example, focused on factors that may affect the unborn child's immune system. Given the elevated rate of childhood asthma and the observation that more than half of children with asthma are diagnosed by the age of 3, researchers have also sought to examine the possible influence of prenatal environments on the developing fetus's risk of developing asthma early in life. Some studies in particular have suggested the possibility of (but not proved) a link between lower-than-normal vitamin D levels in mothers during pregnancy and the development of asthma in their children. More research into why some persons, but not others, go on to develop asthma in the course of their lifetimes is desperately needed. In the case of vitamin D's importance, for example, a clinical trial

Genetic

Related to a gene or a gene product. A genetic trait is an inherited characteristic that is passed from parent to child at conception.

Immune system

The primary defense system of the body. The immune system is responsible for providing protection against bacteria and viruses. The system is composed of the thymus gland, the bone marrow, the lymph nodes (glands), the spleen, and specialized lymphoid tissue located in the intestinal tract.

was scheduled to begin in late 2009 to investigate if adequate maternal vitamin D supplementation in pregnancy leads to a decrease in asthma during the child's first three years of life. The trial is titled, "Maternal Vitamin D Supplementation to Prevent Childhood Asthma (VDAART)"; details are available on the Web at http://www.clinicaltrials.gov/ct2/show/NCT00920621. Vitamin D is also thought to perhaps play a role in asthma symptom severity. John Brehm and colleagues published "Serum Vitamin D Levels and Markers of Severity of Childhood Asthma in Costa Rica" in the May 2009 *American Journal of Respiratory and Critical Care Medicine* and provided evidence of an inverse relationship between vitamin D levels and measures of allergy and asthma severity in Costa Rican children with asthma. The authors also point out that the "Results of some, but not all, epidemiologic studies suggest that vitamin D deficiency is associated with an increased incidence of asthma symptoms . . . higher maternal intakes of vitamin D during pregnancy are associated with decreased risks for recurrent wheeze in young children suggesting that vitamin D may play a role in the development of asthma."

Epidemiologic

Based on the study of populations or of large groups of people.

Clinicians have long noted that certain viral infections seem to be related to the development of asthma in predisposed individuals, both children and adults. Physicians refer to particular "asthmagenic" viruses (such as RSV) that cause typical respiratory infection and symptoms at first, only to leave the patient with an asthma-like condition. Not all infectious agents are viruses, however, and attention has also been directed to other infectious organisms and their possible role in asthma development. Lung infection with a common bacterium (not a virus) called *Chlamydia pneumoniae* (recently renamed *Chlamydophila pneumoniae*) has in particular been suggested (but not proven) as a possible cause of reversible asthma in adults. As of this writing, a clinical trial, AZMATICS:

Asthmagenic

A situation or substance that has the potential to trigger or bring on asthma symptoms, e.g., exercise, exposure to cold air, or response to an allergen.

AzithroMycin/Asthma Trial in Community Settings, is under way at several locations in the United States to attempt to further address the possible link between persistent infection with the bacteria and the development of adult asthma. Details are available at http://www.clinicaltrials.gov/ct2/show/study/NCT00266851.

One of the challenges in studying asthma is that asthma is a heterogeneous condition, which means that it is far from a single disease in terms of symptoms, response to treatment, and associations. Despite their both experiencing episodic cough, wheeze, and shortness of breath, a 6-year-old boy with food allergies, eczema, and year-round asthma does not "have the same asthma" as a 56-year-old woman without any allergy who cannot make it through the New England winters without her inhaler medications, for example. Similarly, a 30-year-old male baker with wheezing and cough due to a type of asthma called occupational asthma (discussed in Question 38) that is related to specific industrial settings and exposures has a different asthma than the aforementioned 6-year-old boy and 56-year-old woman. The development of asthma also reflects the genetic endowment we inherit from our parents. The tendency to develop asthma, particularly in young people, has an inherited basis. If one or both parents have asthma, for example, their child has a greater likelihood of developing asthma as compared to another child whose parents have no personal history of asthma. A study of 344 families residing in Arizona revealed that among children diagnosed with asthma, 6% were from families in which neither parent had asthma, 20% had one parent with asthma, and 60% of children with asthma shared the condition with both parents. Similarly, studies of large populations of twins, comparing asthma and allergy in pairs of identical and fraternal twins, point to an inherited factor required for asthma development. Although it has long been observed

Gene

A unit of heredity made up of a sequence of DNA. Genes are the basic unit of inheritance. They are capable of duplicating themselves each time a cell divides, and genes determine a particular characteristic or trait.

Chromosome

Cellular microscopic structures that contain groupings of DNA. Chromosomes carry genetic information, or genes, in their DNA.

that asthma runs in families, there is no one particular gene known to be responsible for the development of asthma. It appears instead that several genes contribute to an individual's tendency to develop asthma. Still other genes likely influence the disease. Genes located on several chromosomes, such as chromosomes 2, 5, 6, 7, 12, 16, 17, 19, and 20, are important in asthma. Further scientific investigations will hopefully delineate the identification of primary asthma genes, which are those that contribute to the development of asthma in the first place, as well as genes responsible for disease severity (asthma severity-modifying genes), and those determining a response to standard treatments (asthma treatment-modifying genes).

These observations, along with a large body of research findings, have led to the current view that the development of asthma is the result of a complex interaction between a susceptible individual and specific environmental conditions (Figure 2) at a certain point in time.

Gemma's comment:

It's especially important to remember that asthma is tricky: changing weather conditions, humidity holding particles in the air, smoke, and volatile organic compounds all can produce asthma symptoms. In the city where renovations, construction, street repairs, cleaning and heating systems, and blowing stacks can occur at any time, it's important to keep a sharp eye (ear and nose, as well) on the ever-changing environment.

9. What is the relationship between allergy and asthma?

Allergy and asthma are two separate medical conditions, despite the fact that asthma often co-exists with a diagnosis of allergy, especially in children and in teenagers.

Possible Environmental Factors in Asthma Development

The development of asthma reflects a particular genetic or innate predisposition to the disease. In addition, environmental influences have been recognized as significant in the emergence of clinical asthma. The precise interplay between environmental and hereditary factors leading to asthma is still insufficiently understood. It has long been noted that some environmental exposures are associated with progression to asthma while other types of exposures might possibly prevent or delay the development of asthma in susceptible persons. The complex relationships are the subject of ongoing research, at the molecular level, in laboratory animals, and in human populations.

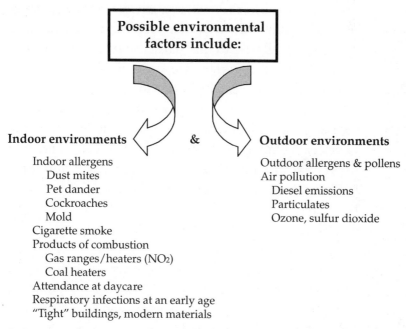

Possible environmental factors include:

Indoor environments & **Outdoor environments**

Indoor allergens
   Dust mites
   Pet dander
   Cockroaches
   Mold
Cigarette smoke
Products of combustion
   Gas ranges/heaters (NO$_2$)
   Coal heaters
Attendance at daycare
Respiratory infections at an early age
"Tight" buildings, modern materials

Outdoor allergens & pollens
Air pollution
   Diesel emissions
   Particulates
   Ozone, sulfur dioxide

Indoor environments play a greater role than outdoor ones in terms of asthma development.

The 2000 report on: *Clearing the Air: Asthma and Indoor Air Exposures* from the Institute of Medicine concludes that there is sufficient evidence to support a causal relationship between asthma development and exposures to dust mites (increased risk of asthma) and environmental tobacco (probably increased risk). Cockroaches, cats, and dogs carry a "maybe" increased risk.

Figure 2   Possible Environmental Factors in Asthma Development.

Exposure to an allergen is harmless to a person who is not allergic to that particular allergen.

Allergy involves our immune systems, which play an important role in asthma as well. An allergy is a very specialized immune response to a specific agent, called an allergen. Examples of allergens include a variety of agents, such as cat dander, cockroach, mold, peanut, penicillin, and ragweed to mention just a few. Most people can play with a cat or eat peanuts, take penicillin for a strep throat infection, or inhale ragweed in late summer in the Northeast and suffer no ill effects at all. That is because they are not allergic to any of those allergens. Exposure to an allergen is harmless to a person who is not allergic to that particular allergen. The person who is allergic to cats or to peanuts, on the other hand, will, upon exposure to cats or peanuts, develop one or more allergy symptoms. Allergy symptoms may arise from different body organs, including the skin (hives), membranes of the eye (conjunctivitis) and nose (rhinitis), the intestines (cramping, nausea, vomiting, diarrhea), as well as the lungs (wheeze).

Asthma, a word derived from the Greek for hard breathing (ἄσθμα) is, as mentioned in Question 1, a disease whose target organ is the lung. A person with asthma may experience intermittent and varying symptoms of cough, mucus production, wheeze, and breathlessness. Part of modern asthma management includes identification of an individual's asthma symptom triggers, with consequent trigger avoidance to any degree possible. A trigger is a stimulus to the development of asthma symptoms, as explained in more detail in Question 41. Some triggers will provoke asthma symptoms in most persons with asthma and are considered universal, whereas other triggers are more personal or idiosyncratic. Cold air and respiratory infections are two examples of universal asthma triggers. That means that the majority of persons with asthma, if exposed to very cold air for a long enough period of time, will likely notice the emergence of some asthma symptoms. They might, when suffering from a significant respiratory infection, also start to develop increased cough and wheezing at night, for instance. Now, take those persons with asthma and expose them to a cat or to ragweed. Those who have no allergy to either cat or ragweed will have no respiratory symptoms at all, whereas those persons with asthma who also happen to be allergic to cats or ragweed, will, if the exposure is of sufficient magnitude, develop allergic symptoms. They may first notice itchy eyes, followed by a runny nose and perhaps wheezing and some cough. The allergen is not a cause of asthma, but rather a trigger (allergic trigger) for the development of asthmatic symptomatology. Exposure to known allergens in a person with both asthma and an allergy can be a symptom trigger for his or her asthma.

Trigger

In the context of asthma, a stimulus to asthma or to allergy. For example, asthma symptoms may worsen when a person with asthma is ill with a viral respiratory infection. In that situation, the infection is considered a trigger for worsening asthma.

Although asthma is different from allergy, a dual diagnosis is far from unusual, especially in children and in adolescents. Published studies indicate that between 60% and 80% of children with asthma also have allergies. An individual of any age with significant allergies is more likely to carry a diagnosis of asthma as compared to someone without any allergy at all. A 12-year-old boy who has been allergic to peanuts or fish since he was a toddler, for example, does not automatically also have asthma. An adult who is allergic to sulfa antibiotics similarly does not inevitably carry an asthma diagnosis. Consider on the other hand, a 17-year-old girl with asthma and an allergy to tree pollen. Each spring, as tree pollen counts rise, she experiences cough, abnormal sensations of chest tightness, and wheezing that requires her increasing and adjusting her inhaled asthma medications. Both the boy and the adult have allergy, and yet they do not have asthma. They each have a diagnosis of allergy alone, whereas

Although asthma is different from allergy, a dual diagnosis is far from unusual, especially in children and in adolescents.

the 17-year-old carries a dual diagnosis of asthma with allergy, with a specific allergen (tree pollen) acting as one of her identified asthma triggers. Her asthma is not caused by her allergy but her asthma symptoms are clearly triggered and exacerbated each spring by her exposure to tree pollens.

Kerrin's comment:

My son developed eczema as an infant. It was particularly bad on his face, and he would develop patches that would not heal no matter what we treated them with, until we finally had to use a steroid cream. He would also occasionally develop hives after breastfeeding, and at 6 months I finally had to wean him because I was down to eating almost nothing for fear that I would induce an allergic reaction, because we could never quite pinpoint exactly what he was allergic to. His eczema eventually went away, but it was replaced with asthma. I was told that it is not unusual for young children with eczema to later develop asthma.

Eczema

An allergic skin condition also known as atopic dermatitis. In babies, eczema often involves the cheeks and diaper area, whereas in older children a distribution behind the elbow creases and the area behind the knees is classic. Eczema can be very itchy and drying.

10. Is asthma preventable?

As mentioned in Question 8, the development of asthma is thought to arise from complex and poorly understood interactions involving a person's inborn genetic characteristics and elements of the environment in which he or she lives, from birth onward. Each of us is endowed with a specific set of genes, inherited from our parents, and there is obviously nothing we can do to alter our genetic makeup. We might thus logically turn our focus to what constitutes the elements of the environment in which we live to see if any preventive measures could prove helpful. An emerging body of scientific evidence suggests that infection with certain common strains of respiratory viruses early in life may predispose a child to develop asthma. Although interesting and a guide for additional research into such viruses and their relationship to asthma, the observation does not carry practical "real life" implications. How, indeed, to avoid a common respiratory virus? There is no feasible way for any of us to avoid catching one!

Over what other parts of our environments might we have more "control"? We can, of course, modify specific exposures in our indoor environments and in particular, in our homes. In 2000, the Institute of Medicine published a report called *Clearing the Air: Asthma and Indoor Air*. It reviewed the available scientific evidence about indoor air exposures and asthma. One aspect of the report looked at those exposures that might represent risk factors for the development of asthma. It concluded that there is sufficient scientific evidence to support a causal relationship between the development of asthma and exposures to house dust mites as well as a strong association between exposure to secondhand smoke (called ETS for environmental tobacco smoke) and asthma in younger children. The ETS exposure included prenatal exposure. Exposure to cockroaches and to the respiratory syncytial virus (RSV) were less clear-cut risks for asthma, but both appeared to increase the risk. Not everyone at an increased risk for asthma will inevitably go on to develop the condition, but it is both prudent and reasonable to decrease or eliminate exposures to known risk factors as much as is possible.

In advising a patient, I would focus on lessening exposure to house dust mites, secondhand smoke (ETS), and cockroaches. I would especially emphasize that it is imperative that any woman who smokes be aggressively counseled and assisted in quitting during pregnancy and beyond. The vigorous anti-tobacco approach should continue after the baby's birth and extend to any other household members who smoke to ensure that the home becomes and remains 100% smoke free. Similarly, pediatricians and allergists often make suggestions in an attempt to modify the emergence of allergies and/or asthma in a child thought to be at increased risk for the development of the disease, based on a family history of either allergy or asthma in a parent or older sibling. They may for instance, advise new parents with asthma to follow special guidelines in caring for their newborn. Recommendations typically concern the baby's diet and environment. For example, an exclusive diet of mother's milk for at least the first 4–6 months after birth appears to delay (but not necessarily avert) the development of allergy and asthma. Similarly, early introduction of solid food is frowned upon in an infant at increased risk for asthma. Certain highly allergenic foods should not be part of a toddler's diet, because of the association of allergy and asthma in youngsters. The foods responsible for most food allergies in children include cow's milk, eggs, nuts, and fish. More specifically, 90% of all allergic reactions to food are caused by eight foods: cow's milk, egg, peanut (peanuts are legumes, not true nuts), tree nuts (such as walnuts, cashews, and hazelnuts), fish, shellfish, soy, and wheat. In addition to dietary guidelines, physicians stress the importance of a smoking ban at home. Some pediatric specialists may advise a bedroom free of dust-collecting items such as draperies, stuffed animals, and wall-to-wall carpeting, and they may recommend encasing bedding in specialized covers (encasements) to reduce dust mite exposure.

Dr. Homer A. Boushey is a world-renowned authority on asthma and a professor of medicine at the University of California, San Francisco. In a recent article in the *Proceedings of the American Thoracic Society* medical journal,

Dr. Boushey recapped recent asthma developments as presented at the 2008 Thomas L. Petty Aspen Lung Conference devoted to asthma insights and expectations. He bluntly addresses the frustrating lack of an effective and accessible means of asthma prevention and elaborates:

It is clear that the lay public ultimately expects the development of a cure for those with asthma and of an effective means of primary prevention for those who do not yet have it. They understand that fulfilling these expectations will require good understanding of the causes and mechanisms of asthma, so they appreciate the need to do research, but they don't want us to take too long about it . . . As for prevention, medical science is seen as almost clueless. We know to advise people to avoid exposure of children to secondhand cigarette smoke, to breast-feed babies for 6 months but maybe not longer . . . But we don't seem to know whether to advise buying two dogs or two cats, to avoid peanuts or eat them early, to send young children to daycare to ensure they contract multiple viral respiratory infections or to treat them with immune globulin for RSV bronchiolitis.

The bottom line is that although experts recommend reducing environmental exposures that have shown to be asthma risks, there is no known intervention at the present that completely prevents the development of asthma.

It is important to note that a child may develop allergy or asthma (or both) even though his or her parents have meticulously followed all of their physician's advice. Neither the child nor the parents are in any way "responsible" for the development of the asthma. If you or your youngster has been diagnosed with asthma, there is no point in resorting to a should have, could have, would have mindset, especially given the fact that there is no proven intervention or behavior that confidently completely prevents

Bronchiolitis

An inflammation of the tiniest bronchial tubes. Bronchiolitis can be secondary to an infection (infectious bronchiolitis), or from a noninfectious cause such as cigarette smoking (smoker's bronchiolitis).

allergies or asthma. Instead, commit yourself to successfully managing your asthma and its symptoms.

Once an individual of any age is diagnosed with asthma, initial treatment concentrates on gaining control of the asthmatic episode and on restoring normal lung function. After the initial treatment goals are met, the major focus of contemporary treatment then emphasizes prevention of symptoms such as breathlessness, chest discomfort, cough, mucus production, and wheezing. One class of asthma medications, referred to as "controller" or "maintenance" medicines, is specifically designed and prescribed to maintain normal lung function and to prevent an exacerbation of asthma—what used to be called an asthma attack (see Questions 12 and 14 for more on this subject). Identification of an individual's asthma triggers and avoidance of exposure to those triggers are, in addition to using controller or maintenance medications, other means of successfully preventing asthma exacerbations. You can read more about asthma triggers in Question 41.

Exercerbation

A flare of disease activity or of disease symptoms. An exacerbation of asthma can be caused by a viral infection, for example, and would lead to increased symptoms of cough, mucus, chest tightness, and wheezing.

Kerrin's comment:

From infancy, my son experienced allergic symptoms. He developed eczema when he was a few months old and would occasionally get hives after he breastfed. He later experienced breathing problems that on three separate occasions escalated to the point where he needed to be hospitalized for around-the-clock breathing treatments. When he was about 2 years old, he was officially diagnosed with asthma. Knowing this, and that he had allergic tendencies but not knowing exactly what they were yet, we decided to keep him away from the highly allergenic foods, such as peanuts and cow's milk. As he got older, we would give him small portions of milk to see if he could tolerate it and he seemed to be fine. Because peanuts are the next hardest

Allergenic

Capable of causing an abnormal (allergic) response in a susceptible (allergic) individual. Some substances are considered to be more allergenic than others, meaning that those substances are known to more frequently lead to allergy symptoms in general.

ingredient to avoid, we decided that we would have him tested for this allergy. Before we even got the chance, he took a bite of a cookie that had either been baked with peanut oil or had touched another item that contained peanut, and he shortly thereafter developed terrible hives. We immediately took him to see a pediatric allergy specialist, who tested him for peanuts, and, sure enough, he had a severe allergy. We were told that the next time he is exposed to peanut, the symptoms could be even more severe and lead to compromised breathing.

11. What is the hygiene hypothesis?

The hygiene hypothesis is a theory that attempts to explain the increased prevalence of allergy and asthma in affluent, industrialized nations. It also strives to elucidate factors that are responsible for the development of asthma in individuals.

The British epidemiologist David Strachan advanced the beginnings of the hypothesis in 1989 after studying the health records of 17,414 British children born during a week in March 1958 and followed up to the age of 23 years. "Hay Fever, Hygiene, and Household Size," published in the November 18, 1989 issue of *The British Medical Journal,* sought to correlate the presence or absence of childhood hay fever and eczema with data on 16 perinatal, social, and environmental factors. The resultant hypothesis proposes that the rising prevalence of asthma and allergic diseases parallels the decreasing prevalence of infections in childhood. Over the last 100 years, urbanization, advances in public health, improved sanitation, and the adoption of cleaner living environments, along with the introduction of antibiotics, have all led to reduction in infectious illnesses in children. During the same period, the occurrence of asthma and allergic diseases has increased. The hygiene

Hygiene hypothesis

A theory that links exposure to dirty environments and to certain infectious agents at specific times in early childhood to a decreased risk for the development of asthma.

Prevalence

In medicine, the total number of cases of a disease diagnosed at a given point in time. Includes all cases, whether the diagnosis is new or more longstanding.

hypothesis links the two observations. The hypothesis suggests that the reduced exposure to "dirty" environments and to infectious agents at a specific point in childhood leads to less stimulation of certain parts of a growing child's immune system. Changes consequently fail to take place in the maturing immune response, and the absence of those changes, in turn, predisposes that child to an increased risk of developing allergies or asthma.

Epidemiologic studies lend credence to the hygiene hypothesis. Exposure to a farming environment, for example, and to farm animals in particular, appears to protect against the development of asthma. Children raised on farms encounter a different range of organisms (animals, viruses, bacteria) than do children raised in industrialized urban centers. Several studies have shown that the children from farming communities have a lessened occurrence of asthma, hay fever, and allergy. Another example that strongly supports aspects of the hygiene hypothesis is provided by the recent work of Dr. Martin Blaser, an infectious disease specialist and prominent researcher who studies *Helicobacter pylori*. *H. pylori* is a bacterium found worldwide; it is usually acquired early in life. *H. pylori* is a cause of recurrent stomach and duodenal ulcers and is associated with stomach cancer in adulthood. With the advent of improved living conditions and of antibiotic therapies in contemporary westernized societies during the 20th century, the rates of childhood infection with *H. pylori* have decreased dramatically. That decrease has occurred against the backdrop of increasing childhood asthma (and allergy) leading to the hypothesis that childhood acquisition of *H. pylori* is associated with reduced risks for asthma and allergy. Further, Dr. Blaser and his colleagues reviewed data collected between 1988 and 1994 from 7663 persons as part of the U.S. Centers for Disease Control and Prevention's third National Health and Nutrition Survey (NHANES) as well as that from 7412 individuals from a NHANES follow-up in 1999–2000. The findings demonstrate a significant correlation between the absence of *H. pylori* infection and early onset asthma in children and teens. The association suggests that acquisition of *H. pylori* in childhood does indeed confer protection from asthma and allergic conditions.

The exact cellular mechanism of how exposures protect a person from developing asthma and allergy is unclear. One possibility is that increased numbers of infections or exposure to farm animals (or pets) might stimulate the child's immature immune system to develop along immunologic pathways that lead away from asthma. Research continues in the area of the hygiene hypothesis. An ambitious and far-reaching, ongoing study in that regard is the GABRIEL study launched in 2006, which seeks to identify the genetic and environmental causes of asthma in the European community. GABRIEL consists of a collaboration among 35 partners at major scientific research institutions across the European community, and has recently added partners from Ecuador, Russia, and Hong Kong. The study investigates the genetics, epidemiology, and immunology of asthma in children and adults across several countries. It also will specifically address the hygiene hypothesis. You can follow the researchers' progress at http://www.gabriel-fp6.org.

Is there an age at which a child's immature immune system needs to be stimulated in a specific way, by certain environmental agents, in order for asthma *not* to develop? If such were the case, specific interventions or medications could perhaps be developed to modify a child's risk of asthma. The hygiene hypothesis remains controversial and represents an intriguing theory that is far from definitive at the present. Asthma practitioners require scientific evidence to validate the theory, and so no clinical recommendations can be advanced right now, based on what remains a very interesting conjecture.

12. What is the contemporary view of asthma, and how does it differ from traditional views?

In the past, asthma was considered a disease principally of airway narrowing, termed *bronchoconstriction*. In the traditional view, bronchial passages encircled by specialized muscle fibers became narrowed (constricted), leading in turn to the development of an "asthma attack." The traditional explanation erroneously emphasized that constriction of the bronchial tubes was the primary, underlying event in asthma. The focus of asthma treatment centered only on reversing the constriction of the breathing passages. Asthma treatment consequently consisted mostly of relief of airway narrowing once symptoms of cough, chest tightness, breathlessness, and wheeze had become established and recognized. Emphasis was placed on treatment of attack symptoms, rather than on preventive measures.

The contemporary perspective on asthma recognizes the importance of bronchoconstriction but assigns it a secondary role. The main "player" or "culprit" in asthma is inflammation. In the modern-day model of asthma, periods of active disease or exacerbation emerge from a background of quiescent periods of remission (Table 5). During an exacerbation, there is increased inflammatory activity in the asthmatic lung. The inflammation, if unchecked, leads to mucous gland stimulation with excess secretions and cough, and to eventual

Constriction

Narrowing, the opposite of dilatation.

Inflammation

Inflammation occurs as a consequence of the release of chemicals called inflammatory mediators from specialized white blood cells.

The main "player" or "culprit" in asthma is inflammation.

During an exacerbation, there is increased inflammatory activity in the asthmatic lung.

Table 5   Asthma: Quiescent vs. Exacerbated

Inactive, Asymptomatic Asthma	Active, Symptomatic, and Exacerbated Asthma
Inflammation is absent (or nearly so), and quiescent	Inflammation is heightened
Air passages (bronchi) are clear of mucus	Mucous gland production increases • leads to cough • leads to secretions • leads to noisy breathing
Air passages are fully "open" (patent)	Air tubes constrict and narrow • leads to bronchoconstriction • leads to wheezing • leads to chest discomfort • leads to breathlessness
Asthma is controlled	**Asthma is inadequately controlled**

bronchoconstriction or airway narrowing. The increased mucus leads to cough. The bronchoconstriction is responsible for symptoms of breathlessness, wheezing, and chest tightness.

A key feature of asthma is a predisposition to increased lung inflammation. Individuals with asthma develop enhanced inflammatory responses in their lungs, a finding that goes hand in hand with the diagnosis of asthma. They are said to have an innate state of lung baseline hyperreactivity, which sometimes is referred to as "twitchy airways," a terminology that is strictly speaking incorrect; airways do *not* twitch! I mention the term as it is (alas) used freely in conversations between physicians and their patients in an attempt to describe the distinctive phenomenon of bronchial hyperreactivity. A specialized lung test, called a methacholine challenge (bronchoprovocation) test (described in Question 29), may be helpful to clinicians when evaluating individuals

Remission

In a medical context, the subsiding of disease symptoms. The disease is still present, but it is undetectable to the patient; it has no symptoms.

Controlling and limiting airway inflammation controls asthma symptoms and leads to normalization of lung function, an excellent prognosis, and a healthy lifestyle.

suspected of having asthma and therefore a state of lung hyperreactivity. The tendency to increased baseline hyperreactivity is likely hereditary. Increased baseline hyperreactivity explains why, for example, the lungs of persons with asthma are more "sensitive" to inhalation of different environmental stimuli such as cold air, strong odors, and cigarette smoke. The presence of bronchial hyperreactivity is of great interest to asthma researchers. It is tempting to speculate about a medication that could modify a person's bronchial hyperreactivity and so reduce the severity of his or her asthma.

The current understanding of asthma as a disease primarily of inflammation, with secondary airway narrowing (bronchoconstriction) as a consequence of an increased inflammatory response, has both research and practical implications (Table 6 and Figure 3). It allows for preventive interventions and for more directed medications. Controlling and limiting airway inflammation controls asthma symptoms and leads to normalization of lung function, an excellent prognosis, and a healthy lifestyle. Prompt treatment of an exacerbation always includes anti-inflammatory medication in addition to

Table 6   The Contemporary View of Inflammation in Asthma

The modern view of asthma emphasizes the all-important role of inflammation.

Contemporary asthma treatment includes:

- Avoiding factors that increase lung inflammation
- Use of medications with anti-inflammatory properties

The traditional perspective erroneously assigned a primary role to airway narrowing, called bronchoconstriction.

Bronchoconstriction is the consequence of a more powerful stimulus: underlying airway inflammation.

When airway inflammation is present, treating the bronchoconstriction in asthma without treating the accompanying inflammatory response is inadequate treatment.

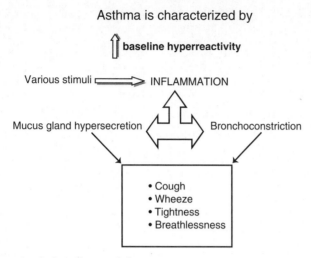

Asthma is characterized by

baseline hyperreactivity

Various stimuli ⟹ INFLAMMATION

Mucus gland hypersecretion   Bronchoconstriction

- Cough
- Wheeze
- Tightness
- Breathlessness

Figure 3   Asthma Characteristics.

specific treatment directed to relief of bronchoconstriction. Recognition of the importance of inflammation in asthma has led to a better understanding of asthma and to the development of more effective treatment.

Asthma exacerbations may occur predictably and inevitably following certain exposures, such as the onset of cold winter temperatures, for example. Some individuals "have an attack" every fall at the change of season and must forgo daily routines, including work and school, or avoid leisure activities. Treatment of established symptoms of an "attack" in the traditional view might include a burst of medication, hopefully in the office setting, but possibly in the hospital. The contemporary view of asthma, however, emphasizes a preventive approach. An individual with asthma and a pattern of worsening symptoms at the change of season would benefit from the prescription of stepped-up anti-inflammatory medication as winter approached. By successfully controlling inflammation and keeping a watchful eye out for the emergence of any early signs and symptoms of disease exacerbation, attacks would be avoided, along with significant lifestyle disruptions.

Recognition of the importance of inflammation in asthma has led to a better understanding of asthma and to the development of more effective treatment.

31

PART TWO

Asthma: Symptoms and Diagnosis

What are the symptoms of asthma?

What is an exacerbation of asthma?

Does wheezing mean that I have asthma?

Are there medical conditions that can mimic
asthma or make it more severe?

How is the diagnosis of asthma established?

What are pulmonary function tests (PFTs), spirometry,
and peak expiratory flow (PEF) measurements?

More . . .

13. What are the symptoms of asthma?

Medical textbooks correctly inform us that "classic" symptoms of asthma are three in number: wheezing, cough, and abnormal sensations of breathing, or dyspnea. If you are studying for a knowledge test, mark those three symptoms on your answer sheet. You will get full credit for the right answers and will surely score an A for your asthma knowledge! Typical asthma symptoms that we see in the office or clinic, on the other hand, represent variations of the big three: an unusual awareness of breathing, uncomfortable breathing, chest pressure or a feeling of chest discomfort, wheezing or noisy breathing, labored breathing, coughing, mucus production, and breathlessness with exertion or effort. Nocturnal symptoms, such as waking from sleep with uncomfortable breathing or wheezing, are indications of less than optimal asthma control and are signs of an asthma exacerbation. Asthma can manifest itself in various modes, from mild to severe. A person with a milder form typically experiences different symptoms at different levels of frequency and intensity than a person with a more severe form of asthma. Children may have a persistent cough (often misdiagnosed as recurrent bronchitis) as their only asthma symptom. Cough is, in fact, the single most common asthma symptom in children. Symptoms of asthma may thus differ from person to person and may vary in an individual over time. Asthma symptoms are usually episodic; symptoms may come and go, and are not necessarily continuously present.

14. What is an exacerbation of asthma?

Asthma is characterized by periods of exacerbations and remission of symptoms, as mentioned briefly in Question 12 (see Table 5). During a remission of asthma, symptoms are well controlled and measurements of lung function

---

Symptoms

What the patient notices, experiences, and reports to his or her treating physician as abnormal or different from usual.

Dyspnea

An abnormal awareness of breathing; a kind of breathlessness.

Nocturnal

Taking place or occurring during the night.

Cough is, in fact, the single most common asthma symptom in children.

Asthma symptoms are usually episodic; symptoms may come and go, and are not necessarily continuously present.

Bronchitis

An inflammation of the lining of the larger bronchial tubes. Bronchitis can be acute, as from infection, or chronic, as in the case of tobacco abuse.

normalize. An exacerbation of asthma, on the other hand, refers to an increase in lung inflammation and represents a period of increased asthma activity. It indicates a flare of the disease. An exacerbation of asthma manifests itself through the development of lung symptoms. Examples of exacerbation or flare symptoms include wheezing, coughing, nighttime lung symptoms, increased mucus production from the lungs, breathlessness or dyspnea, and chest pressure or discomfort (Table 7).

During an exacerbation, measurement of lung function, as indicated by the FEV_1 (and peak flow) will typically show decreasing values. An exacerbation usually develops

Table 7   Asthma Exacerbations: Common Symptoms

Symptoms are what an individual experiences. Physicians and health care providers should always ask patients with asthma to report symptoms. Never ignore new or increasing asthma symptoms.

Breathlessness, with exertion or activity that may progress to occur at rest as an exacerbation progresses in severity

> *"I can't catch my breath; I am out of breath; I need air."*

Cough

> *"I'm just coughing every day, and the cough just won't quit, but I don't have a fever."*

Dyspnea is an abnormal awareness of breathing

> *"I feel my breathing and it is uncomfortable."*

Mucus hypersecretion

> *"I keep bringing up this clear stuff."*

Nocturnal awakenings

> *"Several times this week I wake up at around 2 AM and my breathing is not right."*

Uncomfortable chest sensations, feelings of pressure and/or chest tightness

> *"It feels as if an elephant is sitting on my chest."*

Wheezing

> *"It feels like there's a kitten purring in my chest."*

gradually and begins with mild symptoms. If unchecked, that mild exacerbation will worsen and become more severe. Mild exacerbations, identified early and treated appropriately—perhaps with increased use of inhaled medication—can be nipped in the bud with minimal, if any, disruption of health and lifestyle. More advanced exacerbations, however, may require the use of additional medication, such as steroid tablets. Severe or rapidly progressive exacerbations require hospital-based or emergency department intervention and treatment.

The term asthma exacerbation has supplanted the outdated asthma attack in the scientific and medical literature.

The term *asthma exacerbation* has supplanted the outdated *asthma attack* in the scientific and medical literature. Exacerbation more accurately describes the gradual nature of the buildup in lung inflammation during a disease flare. Some practicing pediatricians, internists, family physicians, and asthma and allergy specialists nonetheless still choose to use the term *asthma attack* in speaking with their patients about asthma. The word *attack*, with its allusion to defensiveness, implies unpredictability, violence, and vulnerability, whereas *exacerbation* emphasizes reversibility and potential transience. I prefer to use the term *exacerbation* throughout this book, just as I do with my patients; it is more accurate and is scientifically accepted. No matter which terminology you use, remember that an exacerbation of asthma, even of the mildest type, should never be ignored or dismissed as insignificant (Table 8).

Treatment of an asthma exacerbation always includes a search for those factors underlying the loss of asthma control. Did wheezing emerge because of a respiratory infection? Were the several missed doses of inhaler medicine the culprit? Could the long wait at the bus stop in the morning in subzero temperature have been a factor? Correct identification of asthma triggers not only allows for a better understanding of your individual

Table 8   Asthma Exacerbation: 10 Key Points

- An exacerbation of asthma is a sign of uncontrolled or poorly controlled asthma.
- An exacerbation of asthma reflects increasing and ongoing lung inflammation.
- An exacerbation of asthma is a significant flare of disease activity; some persons prefer to use the term "asthma attack."
- Never ignore increasing or worsening symptoms such as wheezing, cough, nighttime awakenings, shortness of breath, or chest tightness or pain. Not all symptoms need to be present to define an exacerbation.
- Although asthma exacerbations tend to build up gradually, untreated (or ignored) symptoms can rapidly worsen and may lead to hospitalization, respiratory failure, and even death.
- Lung function measurements including the FEV_1 and PEF usually decrease during an asthma exacerbation.
- Timely and appropriate intervention and response to increasing asthma symptoms will limit their duration and lead to a return to normal baseline lung function.
- Most exacerbations will require the administration of a "burst" of oral corticosteroid anti-inflammatory medication. Some exacerbations may require treatment in hospital.
- Prevention of exacerbations is a major goal of modern asthma management.
- Remember that asthma and its symptoms are controllable with proper treatment.

asthma but also leads to a more proactive approach to managing your asthma, with an emphasis on preventive measures. Learning to increase asthma medicines when specific symptoms of an infection emerge, for instance, may help you prevent a flare or an exacerbation. Another example of proactive asthma treatment might include stepping up appropriate asthma medicine prior to the onset of spring weather if you've been diagnosed with tree pollen allergy and asthma and have had exacerbations in prior years related to blossoming trees.

15. What is a wheeze?

A wheeze is the sound generated when air travels though a breathing passage (airway) that has become narrowed. The narrowing can be due to mucus secretions

Inspiratory

Breathing in.

Expiratory

Breathing out.

Stethoscope

A medical instrument used to amplify and listen to sounds produced by internal organs, such as the lungs, heart, or bowels during a physical examination.

Bronchoconstriction

An abnormal narrowing of the air passages. Bronchoconstriction is a prominent characteristic of asthma and is due to an increased inflammatory response in the lung.

Wheezing is never normal and should never be ignored.

trapped within the airway or to the airway muscles' constriction or tightening around the airway. The airway narrowing due to asthma is reversible. Medications prescribed for asthma help the narrowed airway return to its normal state. A wheeze is best described as a high-pitched whistling sound. Wheezing can occur while breathing in (inspiratory wheezing, during the inspiratory phase of the breath), while breathing out (expiratory wheezing, during the expiratory phase of the breath), or during the entire breath. Asthma is one of several conditions that can cause wheezing, as detailed further in the following question. If wheezing is severe, it can be heard without a stethoscope.

Wheezing in asthma reflects ongoing lung inflammation and airway narrowing, or bronchoconstriction. The sound is generated by turbulent flow through constricted airways. The presence of wheezing in asthma indicates that the asthma is active, and that more intensive and efficacious treatment is warranted. Wheezing is never normal and should never be ignored. If airway narrowing and inflammation are left untreated, there is a real risk of the disease worsening, which can become potentially life threatening.

16. Will I know when I wheeze?

Gemma's comment:

In my teens, I attended a boarding school in northern New York State. I found that in winter I could always develop a noisy wheeze if I opened a window and took big gulps of cold air. The choking cough and noisy breathing that followed was enough to get me excused from what was called winter "sport" (usually shoveling snow off a basketball court!), and that was what I wanted. I didn't think I was sick, just smart. Certainly, I never discussed these symptoms with a doctor, because they served me well: they excused me from unwanted activity. Of course, such wheezes might not have been diagnosed as asthma . . .

Yes, most individuals with asthma can recognize when they are wheezing. They may become aware of the abnormal sound of wheezing as inhaled air travels though narrowed bronchial passages. One might say, "It sounded like a cat purring in my chest." Others may notice an uncomfortable mid-chest pressure. Wheezing should never be ignored or dismissed as unimportant.

The most reliable method for a physician to detect a wheeze is by performing a physical examination that includes auscultation of the lungs with a stethoscope. The physician places the chest piece of the stethoscope on the patient's upper torso—over the front, back, and sides— and listens as air enters and exits the lungs. The patient takes several deep breaths, breathing through his or her mouth, as quietly and smoothly as possible. The physician pays close attention to the symmetry of the breath sounds and to any audible abnormalities, such as wheezing.

In a variant type of adult asthma called cough-variant asthma, wheezing is absent, and a dry, nonproductive cough is the major symptom of asthma. The emergence of wheezing, or of persistent dry cough in the case of cough-variant asthma, is always significant and must be reported to the treating physician. The development of wheezing indicates inadequate asthma control and may herald the beginning of an exacerbation of the disease. The same is true of a cough in cough-variant asthma because the cough is equivalent to a wheeze.

Auscultation

The process of listening to the chest through a stethoscope. Auscultation is performed by the examiner placing a stethoscope on the skin overlying the lungs and having the patient breathe in and out.

17. Does wheezing mean that I have asthma?

No, not necessarily. The to-and-fro movement of air through the lungs and tracheobronchial tree should always be silent. A wheeze is an abnormal sound produced by turbulent flow of air through the lungs. There are many different causes of wheezing The occurrence of a wheeze by itself without any other symptoms is unusual. It is therefore important to note if the wheezing is recurrent or if it is associated with other lung symptoms such as breathlessness, cough, or mucus production.

Medical students learn that not all that wheezes is asthma. Although most people with asthma will at some point experience wheezing, not everyone who wheezes has a diagnosis of asthma (Table 9). Some people who wheeze will turn out to have a lung condition other than asthma, while others will wheeze even though there is no identifiable lung condition and the lungs appear completely normal. The first category includes persons with a cigarette-related lung disease such as COPD, for example. Other lung diseases, such as bronchiectasis or bronchiolitis, can also lead to wheezing. Certain lung

Bronchiectasis

A lung disease that causes abnormal, permanent dilatation of the small bronchiolar air tubes and passages that lead to the lung alveoli. Bronchiectasis causes a wide spectrum of disease.

Table 9   Causes of Wheezing

Asthma
Foreign body aspiration
COPD
   chronic obstructive bronchitis
   emphysema
Bronchiectasis
Lung infections, infectious bronchitis, bronchiolitis, croup
Allergic reaction (severe, anaphylactoid)
Congestive heart failure
GERD (gastroesophageal reflux disease)
Drug induced (beta-blockers)

infections can cause wheezing in completely normal lungs. Some people without any lung disease but who have congestive heart failure can wheeze if they take in too much fluid. Still others might wheeze after a severe allergic reaction, such as to a bee sting, for example. Gastric reflux, called GERD (gastroesophageal reflux disease), is a disease of the digestive system and is an example of a non-pulmonary condition that can mimic asthma. Similarly, vocal cord dysfunction (VCD) syndrome affects the voice box (larynx) and is often confused with asthma. Finally, and especially in children, a wheeze can be caused by a foreign body trapped in the bronchial tree. Young children, in particular, explore the world by putting objects in their mouths. From there, it's a short trip into the breathing passages. A foreign body should be retrieved from the lung passages, usually via bronchoscopy. Medical journals and textbooks have described the successful retrieval of many disparate items, including fish and chicken bones, coins, toy fragments, and even a coffee stirrer.

If you have experienced wheezing, especially on more than one occasion and perhaps associated with other symptoms, consultation with your physician is the appropriate next course of action. Your doctor will be able to ascertain if the wheeze is due to asthma or not and can advise you on what treatments would be indicated for you.

Gastroesophageal reflux disease (GERD)

A condition that, when present, may lead to abdominal symptoms and heartburn and may also significantly worsen underlying asthma. GERD, or more simply reflux, is usually treated with a combination of dietary changes and medicine.

Vocal cord dysfunction (VCD) syndrome

A condition that can be confused with asthma. VCD syndrome's primary disturbance involves the vocal cords and their abnormal tendency to move toward each other (rather than move apart) during inspiration, or breathing in.

18. Why do I usually cough after jogging or running or after participating in sports?

The presence of a persistent cough is always abnormal. There are many reasons why cough may develop. Each one of us has experienced a cough at some point in our

The presence of a persistent cough is always abnormal.

lives, when ill with a respiratory infection or a head cold, for example. Most coughs due to the common cold are short lived and tend to resolve within a month's time. When a cough lasts longer than 3–6 weeks or assumes a particular repetitive pattern, take note. Lung specialists define a chronic cough as a cough that has been present for more than 8 weeks. The majority of individuals with chronic cough who are not cigarette smokers have one of three causes for their cough: asthma, stomach reflux (GERD), or postnasal drip syndrome (recently renamed UACS for upper airway cough syndrome). Cough that regularly occurs with or following aerobic exercise strongly suggests the presence of asthma unless proven otherwise.

Exercise is considered a symptom trigger in all persons with asthma. Exercise does not cause asthma but acts as a stimulus to bronchoconstriction in asthma and leads to increased airway inflammation. In young children in particular, cough with exertion should never be ignored; it may be the tip-off to the diagnosis of asthma since cough is the most frequent symptom of asthma in children.

Sinus

Air-filled cavities within the human skull. Adults have several sinuses, named by location: the frontal, ethmoid, sphenoid, and maxillary sinuses. The sinuses continue to form after birth; consequently, the frontal and sphenoid sinuses are not well developed in children.

Answering the question of why you might be coughing after running or jogging would require an evaluation that should begin with a medical history (including any medication you are taking), discussion of cigarette smoking if applicable, reviewing the chronology of the symptom, and a physical examination with close attention to the sinuses, throat, heart, and lungs. Additional testing might include a chest X-ray (depending on your individual medical history) and pulmonary function testing. Question 26 provides more information on how asthma is diagnosed.

19. Could my lung symptoms be due to a condition other than asthma?

Yes, depending, of course, on what your exact symptoms are. Medical students and physicians in specialty training are taught the skill of differential diagnosis. When reviewing and analyzing a patient's report of symptoms, the physician generates a list of different possible conditions that could theoretically be responsible for the symptoms. That list of possible conditions is called the differential diagnosis. The physician then ranks the possibilities in order of likelihood. The most likely, based on the information available, is listed first. The next step usually involves attempting to confirm, or "rule in" the doctor's initial diagnostic impression by performing specific tests as needed, in addition to history taking and to the physical examination. For example, the differential diagnosis of a persistent, daily, dry cough that lasts more than 2 months in a 22-year-old non-smoking college student in otherwise excellent health might include asthma, UACS (postnasal drip), or GERD, either alone or in combination. The physician would thus initially perform an evaluation for the possibility of asthma and perhaps even prescribe asthma medication. If the results of that initial evaluation were not consistent with asthma and if the student continued to cough despite asthma treatment, then the doctor would turn his attention to the second possibility on the differential diagnosis list: postnasal drip. A trial of appropriate medication might help in deciding if UACS (postnasal drip) were responsible for the underlying cough. If that intervention were unrewarding and cough still persisted, then the physician would turn his attention to the possibility of active GERD. You can tell from the example that elucidating the origin of a chronic cough may require several doctor visits, along with a good dose of patience! You will also recognize the advantage in consulting a clinician skilled in differential diagnosis, one with the expertise and experience to correctly assess the probability of asthma, rather than one who lists all possibilities and tries to rule in or rule out every single one.

Cardiac asthma

An outdated term that refers to the symptoms produced by dysfunction of the left ventricle, the heart's main pumping chamber in a condition known as CHF, or congestive heart failure.

Several medical conditions are well known to mimic asthma (Table 10), which sometimes makes for a challenging differential diagnosis. Vocal cord dysfunction (VCD) syndrome, for example, exhibits symptoms similar to asthma. Specific types of heart disease, such as congestive heart failure, can be mistaken for asthma. Some physicians even use the term *cardiac asthma*, a misnomer, to describe the wheezing sounds associated with congestive heart failure. Similarly, lung diseases

Table 10   Differential Diagnosis of Asthma in Adults

Certain other lung diseases lead to symptoms that share similarities with asthma:
- COPD (chronic obstructive pulmonary disease that includes emphysema and chronic obstructive bronchitis)
- Pulmonary embolus
- A lesion or tumor—benign or malignant—that obstructs a major airway
- Rare lung diseases such as PIE (pulmonary infiltrates with eosinophilia or eosinophilic pneumonia)

Cardiac dysfunction can also mimic certain asthma symptoms.
- CHF (congestive heart failure)

Specific dysfunction of the digestive system can "look" like asthma.
- GERD (gastroesophageal reflux disease)

Disorders of the voice box can be confused with asthma.
- Vocal cord dysfunction (VCD) syndrome
- Laryngeal dysfunction or tumors

Prescription medications can give asthma-like symptoms.
- ACE inhibitor-induced cough
- Beta-blocker-induced wheezing and exertional shortness of breath

other than asthma can be responsible for symptoms suggestive of asthma. Emphysema and chronic obstructive bronchitis can resemble asthma, but a significant history of smoking cigarettes is usually present. Pulmonary sarcoidosis can cause wheezing. Rare lung diseases like obliterative bronchiolitis or eosinophilic pneumonia are also occasionally in the differential diagnosis of asthma-like symptoms. Common medical conditions that lead to symptoms similar to those of asthma are reviewed in Question 23.

20. What is COPD?

COPD is an acronym for the term *chronic obstructive pulmonary disease*. Chronic obstructive pulmonary disease is a descriptive term rather than a single disease, although it usually is used to refer to emphysema or to chronic obstructive bronchitis.

Technically, COPD refers in a general way to several different lung conditions that demonstrate an abnormality on spirometry, a type of pulmonary function test (see Question 28 for more about pulmonary function tests). The abnormality that characterizes COPD is called *obstructive dysfunction*. Several different lung conditions typically exhibit the obstructive dysfunction pattern of abnormality on pulmonary function testing. They include emphysema, chronic obstructive bronchitis, exacerbated asthma, and bronchiectasis. The two first diseases, in particular, share several features. Both emphysema and chronic obstructive bronchitis are associated with cigarette smoking. Both exhibit obstructive dysfunction on spirometry that does not completely reverse with medication, and thus demonstrate a "fixed" or "irreversible" type of obstructive dysfunction. Both cause respiratory symptoms such as breathlessness or

Emphysema

One of the COPD group of lung diseases. Cigarette smoking is a significant risk factor for the development of emphysema.

Chronic obstructive bronchitis

Chronic obstructive bronchitis is the technically correct medical term for the cigarette-related type of COPD that demonstrates obstructive dysfunction on PFTs and that causes symptoms of cough, mucus production, breathlessness, and episodes of wheezing.

COPD

An acronym for chronic obstructive pulmonary disease. COPD refers to several different lung diseases that share similar symptoms and that demonstrate a similar pattern of dysfunction on the spirometry part of PFTs.

cough. Interestingly, emphysema and chronic obstructive bronchitis frequently co-exist, usually in a current or former cigarette smoker.

Partly because emphysema and chronic obstructive bronchitis appear at first glance to be so similar, physicians have taken to using the term *COPD* to refer specifically to either emphysema or chronic obstructive bronchitis, or even to a combination of both. The use of COPD as a kind of shorthand for the smoking associated lung diseases, whether emphysema or chronic obstructive bronchitis, has taken hold among medical professionals as well as the general public, despite disapproval from some linguistic purists.

21. Is COPD related to asthma?

Asthma is a specific lung disease that is different from emphysema and chronic obstructive bronchitis. COPD is often used as a kind of shorthand to describe emphysema, chronic obstructive bronchitis, or a combination of both, as mentioned in Question 20. COPD always refers to diseases that are not asthma. The COPD group of lung diseases is not related to asthma, although emphysema and chronic obstructive bronchitis exhibit similarities to asthma, reviewed in the next answer. Confusion seems to arise under several circumstances. In the first case, COPD can co-exist with asthma, typically in an older adult with a history of cigarette smoking, and both conditions are present together. Secondly, some medical practitioners in a blatant misuse of language use the word *asthma* to refer to the breathlessness characteristic of the COPD group of lung diseases. They tell their patients with pure emphysema or chronic obstructive bronchitis that they have "a touch of asthma" rather than explaining that the symptom of shortness of breath is a fundamental manifestation of the COPD. Finally, COPD and asthma

Spirometry

One of the pulmonary function tests; the most important pulmonary function test in the setting of asthma diagnosis and treatment. Spirometry measures the flow of air from the lungs as a person forcefully and fully exhales from a deep inspiration.

Obstructive dysfunction

A pattern of abnormality detected by pulmonary function testing. Several different lung conditions lead to obstructive dysfunction on spirometry, one of the PFTs. Asthma is one of the conditions that, on testing, demonstrates obstructive dysfunction. A key element of the obstructive dysfunction uniquely seen in asthma is that, by definition, the obstruction (or abnormality) is completely reversible.

COPD always refers to diseases that are not asthma.

are treated with inhaled medications, some of which are effective in both conditions. On occasion, two family members or friends with two different diagnoses may (correctly) be prescribed the same inhaler, and that can lead to all kinds of assumptions.

I am reminded of a 75-year-old in my care; he had smoked heavily and had marked emphysema. He had succeeded in kicking his former cigarette habit, an achievement of which he and I were very proud. He was naturally quite concerned about the emphysema diagnosis. He explained to me that he was particularly troubled about what his prognosis and quality of life would become over time. Over the course of a year, I prescribed several medications for treatment of his emphysema and he would see me in the office every few months for follow-up. On one memorable visit, he arrived in excellent spirits and shared the news that his 21-year-old grandson who had been diagnosed with asthma at the age of 6 was in town and staying over for a weekend visit. On that visit, my patient discovered that he was taking the identical inhaled medication that his grandson used for asthma, and announced grinning from ear to ear, "Well, Doc, I figured out then that you're treating me not only for emphysema, but for asthma, too, and that means my prognosis isn't that bad . . ."

22. What are the similarities and differences between asthma and COPD?

COPD and asthma are lung ailments. Asthma and COPD can both give rise to similar symptoms, and are sometimes treated with the same medicines. Both conditions can lead to variable breathlessness, wheezy breathing, coughing, and mucus production. Some medicines prescribed for the treatment of asthma, such as inhaled β_2

Agonist

A drug that exerts its actions by combining with specific sites (called receptors) in the body. Albuterol, for example, attaches to the lungs' β_2 receptors. By attaching to the β_2 receptors, albuterol exerts its bronchodilatory effects and causes narrowed bronchial passages to dilate or open up.

agonists, corticosteroid inhalers, and theophylline, for example, are also used in COPD treatment. Asthma and the conditions caused by COPD may also demonstrate a similar pattern of abnormality on the pulmonary function test called spirometry. That similar pattern of abnormality is called obstructive dysfunction.

To a pulmonologist involved in direct patient care, COPD and asthma are completely different. The single most common cause of COPD is cigarette smoking. COPD is a disease of mid- to late-adulthood. It is the fourth leading cause of death in the United States, and it is a significant cause of lifestyle limitation reflecting its chronic and progressive nature. COPD affects different sites in the lung than does asthma, involving both the lung tissue and the airways. COPD's obstructive dysfunction on spirometry is "fixed" or "irreversible" as mentioned in Question 20. Asthma has a genetic basis and is often seen in persons who also carry a diagnosis of allergy. It affects all ages and is frequently diagnosed in children. The diagnosis of asthma is compatible with a long and full life and the prognosis is excellent. Asthma targets the lung airways. By definition, the obstructive dysfunction demonstrated on pulmonary function tests in asthma is reversible such that lung function has the potential to fully normalize.

Pulmonary embolus

A clot, usually originating in the leg veins, that becomes lodged in the lung circulation. The diagnosis of pulmonary embolus can be very difficult. Pulmonary embolus leads to a variety of symptoms, which can include breathlessness and wheezing. A large or massive pulmonary embolus is a cause of sudden death.

23. Are there medical conditions that can mimic asthma or make it more severe?

Yes, several medical conditions can mimic asthma. Surprisingly, not all of them are lung diseases! The lung diseases that should be differentiated from asthma include the COPD group (such as emphysema and chronic obstructive bronchitis) and pulmonary embolus, as well as rarer diseases such as eosinophilic pneumonia and pulmonary infiltrates with eosinophilia. A benign or malignant growth (tumor) arising in the major bronchial tubes can also lead to wheezing and shortness of breath and could be confused with asthma. Conditions affecting the upper respiratory system, more specifically, the larynx or voice box, are well-known asthma copycats. Vocal cord dysfunction (VCD) syndrome, along with dysfunction and tumors of the voice box, are good examples.

The non-pulmonary asthma mimics include cardiac diseases, such as congestive heart failure, and digestive diseases, principally reflux and GERD. Finally, certain prescription medications can produce asthma-like symptoms in susceptible individuals. The antihypertensive medicines known as angiotensin-converting enzyme-inhibitors can occasionally give rise to a nagging, dry cough that is easily mistaken for an asthmatic symptom. Beta-blocker medication, used in the treatment of glaucoma and cardiovascular disease, can in some individuals cause wheezing and breathlessness, often indistinguishable from asthma.

Medical conditions such as sinusitis, allergic rhinitis, and GERD can aggravate asthma symptoms, particularly if the co-existing conditions are not addressed and treated appropriately. Obesity and untreated obstructive sleep apnea syndrome (OSAS) may worsen existing asthma, if present. Up to 21% of adults with asthma also have aspirin sensitivity, as explained in Question 37. They will experience severe exacerbations after taking aspirin (or any of the non-steroidal anti-inflammatory class of medication), which must thus be avoided for life. Sulfites, a type of food additive, can precipitate an exacerbation in sulfite-sensitive persons with asthma. In addition to avoidance of known asthma triggers, good asthma management should thus include identification and prompt and effective treatment of any concurrent illnesses (Table 11).

Asthma: Symptoms and Diagnosis

Eosinophilic pneumonia

A rare type of lung disease characterized by breathlessness and elevated eosinophil counts like asthma, but with abnormal X-ray studies, unlike asthma.

Pulmonary infiltrates with eosinophilia (PIE)

A very rare lung disease. PIE can have symptoms that mimic those of asthma. The chest X-rays and chest CT scans are abnormal in PIE, which is one differentiating feature from asthma.

Sinusitis

An inflammation of the lining of sinuses, due most commonly to either infection (viral or bacterial sinusitis) or allergy (allergic sinusitis).

Allergic rhinitis

A manifestation of allergy expressed as nasal symptoms with itching, runny nose, and congestion. When due to seasonal airborne allergens, allergic rhinitis is sometimes referred to as "hay fever" or "rose fever."

Table 11   Control of Factors Affecting Asthma Severity

Any of the nine factors described here may contribute to making your asthma more difficult to control.

Factor	Control Measure
Allergens	Correctly identify specific allergens and address appropriately: avoidance, antihistamine therapy, immunotherapy injections. Epinephrine auto-injectors for emergency use might be prescribed.
Tobacco smoke	Smoking cessation, smoke-free home and work environments
Rhinitis	Directed therapy: nasal sprays (cromolyn, nasal steroids), nasal washes, antihistamines, leukotriene antagonists, decongestants
Sinusitis	Correct diagnosis is important; drainage measures, washes, nasal steroids, antihistamines, and/or decongestants may be prescribed. Antibiotic therapy is reserved for acute bacterial infections.
Gastroesophageal reflux disease, also known as GERD	Dietary manipulations; small, frequent meals; prescription antacid medication. Elevation of the head of the bed may be advised.
Sensitivity to sulfite additives	Sulfite-sensitive asthmatics should avoid all sulfite-containing foods. Common examples are red wine, beer, shrimp, and dried fruits.
Selected medications	Beta-blockers in any form: eye drops (used in glaucoma treatment) as well as pills (used in high blood pressure and heart disease treatment) can cause bronchospasm. "Aspirin-sensitive" persons with asthma must avoid aspirin and the nonsteroidal, anti-inflammatory class of medicines.
Viral respiratory infections	Yearly influenza vaccination should be recommended (unless contraindicated).
Occupational exposures	Importance of a safe workplace environment: proper ventilation, avoidance, and when appropriate, personal protective respirators

24. What is vocal cord dysfunction (VCD) syndrome?

Vocal cord dysfunction (VCD) syndrome, a notorious asthma mimic, was first described in 1983 by doctors from the National Jewish Hospital in Denver, Colorado.

VCD is the result of abnormal paradoxical vocal cord movement. Humans have two vocal cords located in the larynx, or voice box, which is an organ in the upper neck. The vocal cords are crucial to speech and sound production. The two vocal cords come together in a *V*-shaped configuration and are joined at the base of the *V*. The anatomy of the cords permits them to move closer together, closing the *V*-shaped space between them. When you breathe in, the vocal cords assume an even wider *V* shape and spread further apart to allow air into the trachea and lungs. In active VCD, however, the vocal cords close instead of opening normally during inspiration. Because the cords swing together instead of moving apart, the flow of air into the trachea and lungs becomes compromised. Wheezing occurs as air is forced through the abnormally narrowed vocal cord opening. Other symptoms of VCD include a change in voice quality, hoarseness, throat or chest tightness, and difficulty swallowing.

VCD is often misdiagnosed as asthma, especially as difficult-to-control, or refractory, asthma. Clues to its diagnosis include non-response to asthma treatment, a preponderance of throat and voice symptoms, as well as the absence of nocturnal symptomatology that is so characteristic of asthma. VCD can occur in childhood, adolescence, or adulthood, but is more common in people who are in their 20s to 40s. In younger patients, VCD may occur during competitive sports and seems to have an association with a driven or high-achieving personality style. Psychological factors may be important in adults as well. Among adult patients, women predominate, as do female healthcare workers, for reasons that are not understood.

If VCD is suspected, referral to a specialized center familiar with diagnosis and treatment of VCD should be

Aspirin

Aspirin has analgesic and antipyretic properties; it is prescribed to relieve pain and fever. Because of its anti-inflammatory actions, it is also used in the treatment of rheumatoid arthritis and juvenile rheumatoid arthritis, as well as in the treatment of many forms of heart disease.

Inspiration

The action of taking a breath of air into your lungs. The respiratory cycle has two parts: inspiration and expiration.

strongly considered. It is especially important to determine whether VCD is present alone, or whether there is a dual diagnosis of asthma and VCD, as they can occasionally exist together. Treatment of VCD includes discontinuance of any non-indicated medication, particularly steroids. Specialized speech therapy is the mainstay of treatment and is accompanied, when appropriate, by relaxation exercises and psychological support.

25. What is GERD, and why does it affect my asthma?

GERD is an acronym for gastroesophageal reflux disease, a medical condition related to the regurgitation of stomach acid. GERD is very common and is typically manifested as heartburn and indigestion, including a sour taste in the mouth. We all produce acid in our stomach to assist in digestion of the food we eat. The lining to the stomach is unharmed by the presence of acid. When acid refluxes (flows backwards) from the stomach into the esophagus, which is the body's swallowing tube, the vocal cords may become irritated. Hoarseness and a cough similar to throat clearing may ensue. Finally, any acid reaching the uppermost respiratory passages can cause cough and wheeze, similar symptoms to those of asthma. GERD not only mimics asthma symptoms, but also is thought to worsen stable asthma. Nighttime reflux due to GERD can, for instance, contribute to increasing nocturnal asthma symptoms. The good news is that GERD is highly treatable. First-line treatment consists of straightforward dietary and lifestyle modifications, as well as medication to reduce the stomach's acid production. Sometimes measures as simple as avoiding carbonated beverages, alcohol, caffeine, fried and highly seasoned foods; eating frequent, smaller meals; and not eating for 3 hours before bedtime will do wonders for reflux symptoms. Better reflux control may lead to improved asthma control and to reduced asthma symptoms.

26. How is the diagnosis of asthma established?

Gemma's comment:

In my 60s, I had, at different times, two primary care physicians: one whose specialty was gastrointestinal medicine, the other whose specialty was cardiology. In routine interviews, they both asked if I coughed on a daily basis, and of course, I said "yes." Yet neither one suggested that I should see a pulmonologist, and I was not surprised, since I was used to coughing and thought of it as normal. My asthma was diagnosed only when I turned up for a routine visit in the cardiologist's office with a bad cold and a wheeze. In the light of my experience, it's easy for me to believe that asthma is underdiagnosed.

The diagnosis of asthma is often straightforward, but can also be time consuming and elusive. Asthma can manifest differently in different individuals because of its waxing and waning nature, as well as its variability. A physician evaluating a patient with a typical, or textbook, presentation will likely be able to diagnose asthma correctly at the first visit. A patient with variant or atypical symptoms may require repeat visits or specialized diagnostic testing to confirm the suspected diagnosis of asthma. More severe forms of asthma are usually easier to pinpoint and diagnose accurately. Consider some examples in each category. A previously healthy, nonsmoking young adult who reports an episodic history of intermittent wheezing, cough, chest discomfort, and breathlessness with exposure to cold winter air is describing a history typical of asthma. The college student

Asthma can manifest differently in different individuals because of its waxing and waning nature, as well as its variability.

Asthma can be confidently diagnosed when specific symptoms, physical examination findings, and specialized lung test results are present.

Pulmonary symptoms

Symptoms experienced by an individual and related to the lungs and to the act of breathing. Wheezing, cough, breathlessness, and mucus production are examples of pulmonary symptoms.

Some questions may at first sound intrusive, but should nonetheless be answered truthfully.

who sees the doctor because of a nagging cough and who is concerned about chronic or recurrent bronchitis and colds, might actually be asthmatic. Similarly, the teenager who gets "really winded" playing racquetball, and then gets used to coughing for a few hours after each match, could certainly have asthma as well.

Asthma can be confidently diagnosed when specific symptoms, physical examination findings, and specialized lung test results are present. The first step in the evaluation of suspected asthma is a complete detailed medical history, during which the doctor and the patient meet face to face for an in-depth conversation and exchange of information. The patient will describe what symptoms he or she is experiencing, and the physician will ask a series of directed questions regarding lung health, followed by more general health inquiries. In this fashion, the physician will obtain information not only about the patient's specific pulmonary symptoms, but also about the presence or absence of allergies, and other medical or surgical conditions. Other important background information derives from review of the patient's medication history, along with his or her travel, occupational, and social history. Some questions may at first sound intrusive, but should nonetheless be answered truthfully. When I ask a patient if there is wall-to-wall carpeting in the bedroom, or who does the vacuuming, for example, I am far from interested in discussing domestic decorating or cleaning arrangements. Rather, I am gathering facts to help me decide whether an allergic response to the home environment is a possibility. Similarly, when I ask, "Is anyone else at home coughing, too?" or "Is anyone at home a smoker?" I am searching for clues to help me hone in on the correct diagnosis. All conversations between my patients and me are entirely confidential; truthfulness between us is an important part of the successful doctor–patient relationship. Just as I would never think of telling a patient an untruth, so, too, do I count on my patients to provide me with an accurate description or history.

After history taking comes the physical exam. Most lung specialists will perform a directed physical, with special emphasis on the upper respiratory tract (nose, throat, sinuses), lungs, and the skin. One can expect measurement of vital signs, including blood pressure, respiratory rate, pulse, and if necessary, temperature. Inspection, percussion, and auscultation are techniques that examine the lungs. Inspection refers to a visual look. The specialist will check whether both lungs move in and out with each breath, for example. Percussion involves gently tapping on the chest, listening for clues as to whether or not the lungs are full of air. If the lungs are full of air, the tapping will sound resonant. If the lungs are not entirely filled with air, then the tapping will give rise to a dull sound. Auscultation requires a stethoscope. As described in Question 16, the examiner will ask the patient to inhale and exhale deeply and regularly during auscultation. The presence or absence of wheezing is especially significant.

Percussion

The physical examination of the lungs includes a technique called percussion that requires gently tapping on the chest wall and listening to the quality of the sound produced.

After the history and the physical exam are completed, the doctor will begin to generate a list of diagnostic possibilities, called the differential diagnosis, as outlined in Question 19. The doctor's clinical impression rates the possible diagnoses in order of likelihood. It may sometimes be obvious to the physician that asthma is present. A pulmonary function test called spirometry (obtained before and after inhalation of a bronchodilator medicine) is indicated in order to confirm the suspected asthma diagnosis. If spirometry is not confirmatory and if asthma remains high on the list of possible explanations for a patient's symptoms, then additional diagnostic testing is often obtained (Table 12). The additional testing is

Table 12   Tools for Diagnosing Asthma

- History
- Physical examination
- Pulmonary function testing:
  - Spirometry
  - Peak expiratory flow
  - Challenge testing
  - Arterial blood gas
- Blood tests
- Radiographic tests:
  - Chest X-ray
  - Chest CT scan

helpful in excluding alternative diagnoses and in determining if asthma is the correct diagnosis in spite of the spirometry results.

27. What diagnostic testing is used to diagnose asthma?

The most helpful diagnostic tests for suspected asthma are pulmonary function tests, often referred to as PFTs (discussed in Question 28), and the single most important PFT, both for asthma diagnosis and for follow-up, is spirometry. Other useful medical tests include blood tests and X-ray studies. Additional, more specialized studies may be obtained depending on the clinical picture. An example of a specialized study is skin-prick testing for suspected allergy. Blood tests are valuable in getting an overall picture of a person's health, as well as in excluding other diagnoses. Assessment of immune function and allergies, for example, can be performed in part via blood testing. X-ray studies include conventional chest X-rays, as well as three-dimensional chest CT (computerized tomography) scans. Chest X-rays and CT scans provide information about the anatomy or structure of the lungs and larger breathing passages. In quiescent, controlled

CT (computerized tomography) scan

A three-dimensional imaging technique that provides very precise anatomic detail using X-ray technology. Images of the sinuses and lungs produced by CT scanning provide physicians with accurate information about how those structures look.

asthma, the chest X-ray should be entirely normal. The same is true of the chest CT scan. During an exacerbation, however, the lungs' appearance on an X-ray may suggest what radiologists call hyperinflation, and the CT might reveal air-trapping. Both findings reflect the uneven lung filling and emptying when breathing occurs through inflamed, constricted air tubes.

Magnetic resonance imaging, scanning, and positron emission tomography scanning, while useful in other types of lung diseases, are not required in diagnosing asthma. The same is true of nuclear medicine scans, such as ventilation-perfusion scans and gallium scans.

28. What are pulmonary function tests (PFTs), spirometry, and peak expiratory flow (PEF) measurements?

Pulmonary function tests (PFTs)—as the name implies—are tests designed to measure and assess lung function (Table 13). PFTs were originally research tools, available only in specialized academic hospital centers. They are now widely available and are frequently performed because of their usefulness in the diagnosis and treatment of asthma. Keep in mind as you read this answer that the lung function abnormalities seen in active asthma on PFT testing are, by definition, reversible.

The term *PFTs* is used to collectively describe several different specific tests of lung function. Spirometry is the single most useful of the PFTs when it comes to asthma diagnosis and treatment. Spirometry, in turn, includes two important subtests. The first is called the peak expiratory flow, abbreviated PEF. The second is the FEV_1, the forced expiratory volume in 1 second. Measurements

Hyperinflation

Lung overdistention; sometimes used interchangeably with air trapping, as air trapping results in hyperinflation. Uncontrolled or poorly controlled asthma may lead to hyperinflation, which should abate and reverse with treatment.

Pulmonary function tests (PFTs)

Tests that include the measurement of lung volumes, spirometry, diffusion, and sometimes ABGs.

Keep in mind that the lung function abnormalities seen in active asthma on PFT testing are, by definition, reversible.

Spirometry is the single most useful of the PFTs when it comes to asthma diagnosis and treatment.

Table 13   Pulmonary Function Tests

PFTs were originally designed for physiological lung research. No longer simply a specialized research tool, PFTs help clinicians establish the diagnosis of asthma, and help answer practical questions about disease management and treatment. Items in **boldface** print are PFTs used in the NAEPP's asthma classification and treatment guidelines.

Spirometry (includes **FEV$_1$** and **peak flow PEF**)

How severe is your asthma?

How active is your asthma?

How well controlled is your asthma?

Is additional medicine likely to help?

Measurement of Lung Volumes

What is the biggest volume of air your lungs can contain?

Are you using the most efficient amount of air to breathe?

How severe is your asthma?

Measurement of Airway Resistance

How severe is your asthma?

Measurement of Diffusion

Abnormal in severe exacerbations

Measurement of Gas Exchange or Arterial Blood Gas

Affected in severe exacerbations

Bronchoprovocation Studies

Could asthma be the diagnosis, even though all other above PFT results are entirely within normal limits?

Peak expiratory flow (PEF)

Part of the several different measurements obtained during the spirometry portion of pulmonary function tests.

of PEF and FEV$_1$ are thus parts, or subtests, of the spirometry portion of the PFTs. The availability of inexpensive, highly portable, and easy-to-use peak-flow monitors makes it possible for every person with asthma (even children) to measure his or her peak flow at home on a daily basis in order to monitor asthma activity. FEV$_1$ measurements, on the other hand, require the use of a spirometer, which is more costly, requires special maintenance, and is not presently advised for home use. Self-monitoring of PEF allows a person with asthma insight into his or her condition and permits an assessment of asthma control. Both PEF and FEV_1 play a pivotal role in the National Asthma Education and Prevention Program's (NAEPP's) asthma diagnosis, classification, and treatment guidelines, which are further explained in Questions 32 and 33.

To perform spirometry and PEF, the patient is first asked to take a deep breath of room air. Then, that biggest single breath is forcefully and rapidly exhaled into a mouthpiece connected to the spirometer or peak flow meter. The maneuver is repeated several times during testing to ensure accurate and reproducible values. The spirometer measures the exhaled lung volume, as well as the flow of air through the mouthpiece for the time that exhalation takes place. The spirometry measurements are recorded by the spirometer and are printed out and graphed for review and future reference. Each individual patient measurement is compared to a predicted value. The predicted values for pulmonary function tests are based on three variables: age, height, and gender. Predicted values are different for a 21-year-old, 6-foot-tall man than for a 5-foot-tall, 64-year-old woman. It follows that the PEF value (and the FEV_1) that would be considered within normal limits for a short, older female with asthma would be abnormally low if obtained by a tall, adolescent male with asthma, even though they both had asthma.

Because asthma is characterized as a disease of lung emptying, exhalation time is abnormally prolonged in symptomatic asthma. Anyone with active asthma who attempts to blow out all the candles on a birthday cake with one single mighty blow of air knows about impaired lung emptying firsthand! Depending on the degree of asthma and other factors, such as how much airway narrowing, or

---

FEV_1

Forced expiratory volume in 1 second, which is a subtest of the spirometry portion of the pulmonary function tests. Both the FEV_1 and a second measurement, the FEV_1/FVC ratio, are used to diagnose asthma. Measurement of the FEV_1 is used to assess asthma control and to follow response to treatment.

Exhalation

The action of breathing air out of your lungs, also called expiration. The respiratory cycle has two parts—inspiration and expiration.

bronchospasm, is present, full exhalation during spirometry might last as long as 14 seconds rather than the normal 5 to 6 seconds. The FEV_1 and PEF values reflect the efficiency and status of lung emptying, and thus provide information about how a person with asthma's lung function is affected by his or her condition.

The FEV_1 measures the amount (volume) of air that is exhaled in the first second of forceful exhalation during spirometry as you breathe out as hard and as fast as you can after you have taken in a deep breath. When asthma is poorly controlled, it takes longer than predicted for the lungs to fully empty. Since the total exhalation time is prolonged in symptomatic or inadequately controlled asthma, it follows that the amount (volume) of air exhaled during the first second of that exhalation is lower than predicted. The FEV_1 decreases in symptomatic or poorly controlled asthma. With treatment, the lungs empty more efficiently, and the FEV_1 value returns to a normal range. When asthma is suspected, spirometry is performed before and after inhalation of a short-acting bronchodilator medication to look for the normalization of the FEV_1—a phenomenon called reversibility. The most up-to-date guidelines from the third *EPR* (*Expert Panel Report*) of the National Heart, Lung, and Blood Institute define a 12% or greater increase in a person's baseline FEV_1 on spirometry after use of a bronchodilator as a significant response.

The FEV_1 decreases in symptomatic or poorly controlled asthma.

When active or exacerbated asthma prolongs exhalation, flow of air through narrowed air passages becomes reduced. Spirometry in active asthma also reveals reduced flow rates. The peak flow is the single greatest value of flow measurement that occurs as the lungs start to empty. Peak flows reflect the flow of air through the larger, so-called conducting airways in asthma. Peak flow generally tracks asthma activity. Monitoring peak flow at home allows for comparison of a person's predicted PEF, with his or her actual personal best measurements obtained when the asthma is well controlled, as explained in Question 28. Home-based PEF monitoring can then help identify even a mild exacerbation and guide medication adjustment up or down, depending on how the PEF value fluctuates from the personal best. Self-administered PEF measurements over time are a component of asthma action plans described in more detail in Question 39.

A peak-flow meter is an easy-to-use device designed to help you assess the degree of your asthma control. Persons who have moderate or severe persistent asthma, persons with a history of severe exacerbations, and persons who have difficulty perceiving when their asthma worsens are most likely to benefit from self peak-flow monitoring. Monitoring long-term, daily peak-flow measurements detects early changes in asthma control that require an adjustment in treatment and helps gauge the responses to those treatment changes. Asthma self-monitoring should be neither a bother nor a nuisance. On the contrary, daily home peak-flow monitoring has been shown to improve asthma control, reduce exacerbations, and decrease absences from school and work. Using a peak-flow monitor may also increase your confidence as it helps you learn how to optimize asthma control and achieve greater mastery over your asthma. Most children can accurately measure their peak flow under adult guidance starting at about 6 years of age. Peak-flow monitoring also allows for objective decisions about modifying your asthma regimen based on information contained in the written asthma action plan your physician has provided.

If your physician gives you a prescription for home peak-flow monitoring, you will be asked to determine your personal best value based on measurements obtained when you feel well and are symptom-free. An asthma action plan provides instructions on what asthma medication to take as the peak-flow value falls into one of three zones labeled green, yellow, or red. The green zone includes peak-flow measurements in the range of 80–100% of your personal best. Yellow corresponds to peak-flow measurements in the range of 60–80% of the personal best value. The red zone includes all peak flow values below 60% of your best. Peak-flow measurements in the red zone indicate that your asthma is poorly controlled, and that you will need to either contact your physician, proceed to the emergency room, or both.

29. What is a methacholine challenge (bronchoprovocation) test?

Methacholine challenge test

A type of bronchoprovocation test. It is a specialized pulmonary function test used in the evaluation of suspected asthma, when the diagnosis is otherwise uncertain.

Bronchoprovocation test

A specialized pulmonary function test that correlates with baseline hyperreactivity (BHR) and that can be helpful in the diagnostic evaluation of suspected asthma.

A methacholine challenge test is a diagnostic test used in the evaluation of suspected asthma when reversibility is not demonstrated on initial spirometry. The methacholine challenge is also used for research purposes to study airway hyperreactivity. It is one type of a class of specialized tests called bronchoprovocation tests. Cold-air exercise tests are another example of a bronchoprovocation test.

A bronchoprovocation test might be ordered in the evaluation of suspected asthma. It is not considered a routine test. Consider a scenario where a patient describes subtle symptoms suggestive of asthma. Spirometry (before and after bronchodilator) and other pulmonary function testing are entirely normal. History, physical examination, blood tests, and X-rays fail to reveal an alternative diagnosis or medical explanation for the reported symptoms. The bronchoprovocation test is then indicated to further evaluate for the possibility of asthma. It is an extremely powerful test for eliminating or "ruling out" asthma. In other words, if the test is negative, then asthma is not present. However, if the test is positive *and* if the symptoms correspond, then the patient likely has asthma. People with asthma demonstrate an increased sensitivity to the inhalation of methacholine and therefore obtain a "positive" test result. The converse statement is not true: Although everyone with asthma has a positive result on methacholine testing, not everyone demonstrating a positive result on methacholine testing will have asthma.

The actual methacholine challenge test is usually performed in a hospital pulmonary function lab. The test requires obtaining a baseline spirometry measurement and then repeating spirometry after inhalation of higher and higher concentrations of methacholine. The baseline spirometry values should be normal, which is why the challenge test is indicated. If the spirometry measurements remain close to baseline values after inhalation of increasing doses of methacholine, the test is said to be "negative," and asthma is effectively ruled out. If, on the other hand, the spirometry values decline significantly after the methacholine inhalation, or if wheezing or other symptoms develop, the test is reported as "positive." The testing immediately stops at that point, and an inhaled, short-acting bronchodilator is promptly administered to relieve symptoms and to reverse the abnormal lung function.

30. What is arterial blood gas (ABG) sampling?

When a physician needs information on how efficiently a patient's lungs are functioning, an arterial blood gas (ABG) can provide the answer. The ABG is a blood test. Performance of a routine blood test requires blood taken

Arterial

Related to one or more arteries. The body's arterial circulation leaves the heart via a major artery named the aorta.

ABG

An acronym for arterial blood gas. The body's arteries carry oxygen-rich (O_2-rich) and carbon dioxide-poor (CO_2-poor) blood to our organs and tissues. The ABG assesses how much O_2 and CO_2 are in the arterial system, which is a reflection of the efficiency and function of the respiratory system.

Respiration

The act of breathing in (inspiration) and then out (expiration). Also refers to the process whereby the lungs exchange gases, more specifically, oxygen (O_2) and carbon dioxide (CO_2) at the level of the alveolus and the alveolar-capillary membrane.

Respiratory failure

A state or illness in which the lungs become incapable of respiration. They become unable to provide the body with needed oxygen and cannot rid the body of accumulated carbon dioxide and metabolic waste products.

from a vein, often from the area near the elbow crease. For an ABG test, however, blood is drawn from an artery instead of a vein, and it is analyzed immediately for oxygen (O_2) content, carbon dioxide (CO_2), and pH, a measure of acidity. The radial artery in the wrist is a frequent site for ABG sampling. The ABG gives information about the arterial blood's oxygen and carbon dioxide content, as well as the blood's acidity. Because the lungs are responsible for the extraction of oxygen from the outside air as well as for the removal of carbon dioxide, analysis of the artery sample for those gases indicates how well the lungs are functioning.

The main function of the respiratory system is to carry out respiration (the exchange of O_2 for CO_2, as described in Question 6). Respiration provides the body's vital organs with oxygen and allows for removal of accumulated waste products, primarily acid. After the blood supply passes though the lungs and picks up oxygen, it becomes oxygen (O_2) rich and carbon dioxide (CO_2) poor. The oxygen-rich blood is then pumped by the heart to the entire body—via the arteries—in order to supply organs with needed oxygen.

Although an ABG is not a routine test in outpatient asthma management, it is frequently used in intensive care settings. If a person is suffering a severe asthmatic exacerbation, the ABG will reveal decreased oxygen and carbon dioxide. If the asthma worsens further, carbon dioxide may rise, and the pH will drop, indicating a dangerous buildup of acid. Such a scenario may indicate life-threatening asthma. If such is the case, respiratory failure will ensue from continued carbon dioxide accumulation and oxygen deprivation; treatment includes life support with a ventilator. Patients on ventilator assistance may require frequent ABG monitoring to assist physicians in selecting optimal ventilator settings and to ensure adequate oxygen delivery to vital organs.

31. What is bronchoscopy?

Bronchoscopy is a lung procedure that allows the physician to look directly into the bronchi and to obtain samples or biopsies of any abnormalities found in the bronchial tree. Bronchoscopy is said to be diagnostic when it is carried out to assist physicians in investigating a lung abnormality. A bronchoscopy is therapeutic when performed to remove excess lung secretions or to retrieve aspirated (inhaled) foreign bodies. There are two types of bronchoscopes (the instruments used to perform bronchoscopy): flexible bronchoscopes and rigid bronchoscopes.

Flexible bronchoscopy is also called flexible fiberoptic bronchoscopy, or FOB. Pulmonologists perform FOB, as do thoracic (chest) surgeons. FOB is usually performed with the patient sedated but breathing on his or her own. The bronchoscopist passes the bronchoscope instrument (or scope, for short) through the nose or the mouth, through the vocal cords, and into the trachea. From there, the bronchoscopist can enter and visually inspect the main bronchi and all narrower divisions. The scope enters the lung passages the same way air does. The scope has a light at its tip, as well as a channel, through which the bronchoscopist can inject local numbing medication, pass biopsy tweezers, and suck up any secretions. FOB is often used diagnostically in the investigation of masses or abnormalities seen on chest X-ray studies.

A rigid bronchoscopy is always performed in the operating room by a thoracic (chest) surgeon with the patient unconscious under anesthesia. The rigid bronchoscope is

Ventilator

A machine that provides respiratory support to failing lungs. Respirators can provide breaths and oxygen to patients who are critically ill. They can also be used to support breathing in a nonhospital setting. Respirator machines, or respirators, are similar, and the terms are interchangeable.

Bronchoscopy

A procedure that allows a lung specialist to visually inspect the lungs' breathing passages (bronchi) and to obtain specimens or biopsies of any abnormalities.

Flexible bronchoscopy

A type of bronchoscopy performed with a specialized fiberoptic instrument called a flexible bronchoscope.

Pulmonologist

A physician specialist with extra training and qualifications in the diagnosis and treatment of the different lung diseases.

Rigid bronchoscopy

A type of bronchoscopy performed with a specialized surgical instrument called a rigid bronchoscope. Rigid bronchoscopy requires general anesthesia and is indicated under different circumstances than flexible bronchoscopy.

Bronchial thermoplasty

An emerging treatment option for refractory, steroid-resistant asthma. It is a minimally invasive outpatient procedure performed through a bronchoscope and targets airway smooth muscle with radio-frequency generated heat.

Bronchoscopy is not routinely performed in the care of someone with asthma.

larger and less maneuverable than the flexible scope. It is considered superior to the flexible scope in two specific settings: when dealing with bleeding within the lung, and when retrieving larger aspirated (inhaled) foreign bodies. It also allows for the placement of bronchial stents in specialized circumstances. Most rigid bronchoscopies are indicated for therapeutic purposes.

Bronchoscopy is not routinely performed in the care of someone with asthma. Rare situations involving very severe asthma, when marked accumulation of mucus extensively blocks the bronchial passages, can require bronchoscopy to remove the thick, obstructing mucus plugs. A novel approach to treating persons with the most severe forms of asthma, bronchial thermoplasty, is currently undergoing a multinational clinical trial (as reviewed in Question 72) and is a procedure performed through a flexible fiberoptic bronchoscope directly targeting the airway smooth muscle.

Having well-controlled asthma is not a contraindication to undergoing bronchoscopy if it is required for evaluation of another (non-asthma) lung condition. It is important that a patient's asthma be quiescent and inactive when the bronchoscopy is performed. In particular, if a person scheduled to undergo bronchoscopy is wheezing, the procedure should be cancelled and the wheezing brought under control before proceeding with the test.

PART THREE

Asthma: Classification and Variants

What is the National Asthma Education and Prevention Program (NAEPP)?

What is cough-variant asthma?

What is the asthmatic triad?

What is occupational asthma?

What is an asthma action plan?

Why should I take asthma medicine if I feel fine?

More . . .

32. What is the National Asthma Education and Prevention Program (NAEPP)?

The National Asthma Education and Prevention Program, or NAEPP, was founded in March 1989 to address the growing problem of asthma in the United States. Although much was understood about asthma itself, treatment and outcomes were clearly suboptimal, especially when viewed from a national perspective. The NAEPP's primary goal is to improve asthma care in the United States. Its focus is education—to teach health professionals, asthma patients, and the general public about asthma. The program strives to improve the quality of life for those with asthma and hopes to decrease asthma-related morbidity and mortality. The NAEPP is administered and coordinated by the U.S. Department of Health and Human Services' National Institute of Health's National Heart Lung and Blood Institute (NHLBI).

The NAEPP's coordinating committee commissioned a panel of medical experts to review the scientific asthma literature in order to improve the clinical management of asthma in the United States and to stimulate additional research on asthma. Its landmark report, the *Expert Panel Report (EPR): Guidelines for the Diagnosis and Management of Asthma* first appeared in 1991. Since then, updated guidelines for diagnosis and treatment of asthma have been published, reflecting the tremendous amount of new information about asthma. A follow-up *Expert Panel Report (EPR-2)* came out in April of 1997. In June 2002, the NAEPP committee added refinements to the 1997 document leading to the *Expert Panel Report: Guidelines for the Diagnosis and Management of Asthma–Update on Selected Topics 2002*. The third and current *Expert Panel Report (EPR-3)* was finalized and then posted online in August 2007. All 440 pages of the *EPR-3* report are available for free

Morbidity

A measure of illness in a given population. The morbidity rate from a disease is defined as the proportion of people affected by that disease per year, per given unit of population.

Mortality

A measure of illness; the rate of death from a disease in a given community or population at a precise point in time. The yearly mortality rate from a disease is defined as the ratio of deaths due to that disease, to the total number of persons in that community or population.

reading and downloading via the Internet (http://www.
nhlbi.nih.gov/guidelines/asthma/asthgdln.htm). Print
copies may be ordered from the NHLBI educational
Materials Catalogue for a small fee from NHLBI
Information Center, P.O. Box 30105, Bethesda, MD
20824-0105.

A key component of all the NAEPP's asthma treatment guidelines is the classification of asthma into four
separate categories based on asthma symptoms, pulmonary function test (FEV_1) values, and disease severity.
An individual with asthma will fall into one of the four
groups at the time of the initial assessment of his or her
asthma severity. Interestingly, that person's classification
may change over time depending on how effectively the
disease and its symptoms become controlled. Patients at
any level of severity can also experience exacerbations,
which also can be mild, moderate, or severe in intensity. The accurate classification of a person's asthma
severity at the time of diagnosis and ongoing follow-up
evaluations of disease control as treatment proceeds is
part of the NAEPP's effort to ensure better care for
persons with asthma of all ages. The NAEPP recommends specific medications and interventions for each
level of asthma severity.

The *EPR-3* update emphasizes assessment of asthma
severity (as in the prior reports) at the time of asthma
diagnosis and adds a complementary formal assessment
of the degree of asthma control obtained through treatment over time. The emphasis on asthma control and
on monitoring the response to therapy are new features of
the 2007 guidelines. The latest NAEPP report presents
updated treatment recommendations based on both the
initial asthma severity rating and the response to ongoing
treatment. The report emphasizes that lung function

Asthma: Classification and Variants

measurements (FEV_1), the frequency and intensity of symptoms, and any functional limitations should be included in the assessment of the degree of asthma control (Table 14). The report advocates a six-step approach to the pharmacologic management of asthma and provides detailed treatment suggestions based on severity, control, and age. The *EPR-3* further separates persons with asthma into three groups for purposes of assessment and asthma treatment: children younger than 5 years of age, children between the ages of 5 and 11 years old, and people who are 12 or older. Within each of those age-related categories, it makes specific treatment recommendations for each level of asthma severity/control and outlines specific medicines for each of the six steps of asthma treatment. Patient education and the development of a partnership between the treating team of healthcare professionals and the patient and his or her family remains an essential component of asthma care as envisaged by the *EPR-3*.

Table 14   Know Your FEV₁

- FEV_1 stands for the **f**orced **e**xpiratory **v**olume in **1** second.
- The FEV_1 is the amount (volume) of air that you forcefully breathe out in the first second after taking a maximal, deep breath.
- Since the FEV_1 is a volume of air, it is expressed in liters.
- The FEV_1 is measured during a spirometry test, which is a test of lung (pulmonary) function. It is a useful test in asthma diagnosis and treatment.
- Be sure to ask your asthma doctor what your measured FEV_1 is.
- Your FEV_1 will be compared to a predicted "normal" FEV_1 value; your measurement can then be expressed as a % of predicted.
- A predicted FEV_1 is based on age, height, and gender. The FEV_1 peaks in young adulthood, and normally decreases with aging; taller persons have bigger predicted FEV_1 than shorter people, and men's FEV_1 are greater than women's.
- Your FEV_1 should be normal—greater or equal to 80% of predicted—when your asthma is controlled.

33. What are the classifications of asthma severity and control according to the NAEPP?

Once asthma is diagnosed, the next step is to determine its severity in order to guide therapy. The NAEPP's third *Expert Panel Report* (*EPR-3*) bases its classification of asthma on the frequency of asthma symptoms, the frequency of nighttime awakenings from asthma, how often a short-acting inhaled β_2 (SABA) bronchodilator is required for symptom relief, the extent that asthma interferes with normal activities, and measurement of lung function (FEV_1). Based on those clinical features, a person's asthma will fall into one of four categories: intermittent asthma, mild persistent asthma, moderate persistent asthma, or severe persistent asthma. Tables summarizing the NAEPP's classification adapted from the *EPR-3* are included in Appendix 2.

A person who is experiencing daily wheeze and cough and who is waking up every other night with asthma symptoms falls into a moderate persistent asthma severity classification, for example. His or her asthma is not well controlled and treatment is unequivocally indicated. All persons with asthma should always be prescribed a short-acting, inhaled β_2 bronchodilator (SABA) for quick symptom relief. To continue with our example, the newly diagnosed individual with not-well-controlled asthma (to use the terminology suggested by the *EPR-3*) needs additional therapy including anti-inflammatory medication, ideally an inhaled corticosteroid (see Question 54 for more about medications used in asthma treatment). The goal of treatment is to obtain control of asthma, stepping up medicine if needed. The *EPR-3* defines three categories of asthma control: well-controlled, not well-controlled, and very poorly controlled.

Physicians and patients alike must be able to recognize good asthma control. Studies have revealed that both groups tend to overestimate the extent of asthma control at the same time that they underestimate the severity and the significance of ongoing asthma symptoms. Patients with asthma too often put up with or simply adapt to having some degree of uncontrolled asthma. They should not accept frequent symptoms of cough, breathlessness, wheeze, or discomfort as normal, nor should they consider it acceptable to have to use their short-acting, quick-relief inhaler two times or more a week. They should never assume that activity limitation is a fact of life. Physicians and caregivers who fail to recognize that a person's asthma is not well controlled will miss a crucial opportunity to prescribe appropriate medications for their patient.

The *EPR-3* emphasizes that the major components of asthma control assessment include how frequently symptoms are present by day, how many nighttime awakenings occur in a week, how often a short-acting, inhaled β_2 bronchodilator medication is required for symptom relief, measurement of lung function (FEV_1), and the frequency and severity of exacerbations (Table 15). The goal of well-controlled asthma is attained when a person with asthma (aged 12 years and older) experiences few or no asthma symptoms (no more often than twice a week), has minimal nighttime awakenings from asthma (no more than twice a month), has no interference with his or her daily activities and routines, and has no need to use a short-acting, quick-relief inhaled β_2 bronchodilator medicine more often than twice a week. Lung function should be close to normal as indicated by an FEV_1 value or PEF value of 80% of predicted. Well-controlled asthma should lead to no more than one exacerbation during a year. Once asthma

Well-controlled asthma should lead to no more than one exacerbation during a year.

becomes well-controlled, the *EPR-3* advises consideration of stepping down asthma medications to adjust the medicine to maintain control with minimal dosages and potential side effects.

34. Are there other ways of classifying asthma besides that of the NAEPP?

Yes, several alternative classifications have recently been developed. They all acknowledge the fact that NAEPP classifications have been extremely useful in guiding asthma care and treatment over the years and have been widely used by practicing physicians in daily patient care.

In May 2006, a task force sponsored by the National Heart, Lung, and Blood Institute; the American Thoracic Society; and the American Academy of Allergy, Asthma, and Immunology unveiled a classification designed specifically for purposes of asthma research. The joint effort divides all asthma into four categories (or phenotypes): infection-induced asthma, allergic asthma, nonallergic asthma, and aspirin-sensitive asthma. Of the four classes, allergic asthma tends to begin early in life and is undoubtedly the most common, affecting up to 88% of all persons with asthma. Infection-induced asthma occurs in children and adults. Nonallergic asthma is more common in adults and occurs more often in women. Aspirin-sensitive asthma phenotype, a more unusual variant of asthma, affects no more than 5% of children with asthma and is more of a concern in adult age groups. The American Thoracic Society believes that the four-phenotype asthma classification system will "enhance interpretation of study findings, promote appropriate comparisons among studies, and facilitate genetics research." Time will tell how useful the tool will be.

In 2006, the Global Initiative for Asthma, or GINA, announced the release of its Global Strategy for Asthma Management and Prevention. GINA, formed in 1993, works with healthcare professionals worldwide to reduce asthma prevalence, morbidity, and mortality. GINA is committed to presenting recommendations for asthma management based on the best scientific information available, worldwide. It began as a collaborative effort between the U.S. National Heart, Lung, and Blood Institute (NHLBI) and the World Health Organization (WHO). GINA comprises networks of individuals and organizations committed to asthma care. It maintains a Web site at http://www.ginasthma.com. If you are familiar with World Asthma Day, held on the first Tuesday in May yearly since 1998, you may already know that GINA is its sponsor. The 2006 GINA guidelines supplanted earlier GINA statements and presented a new, easy-to-implement classification of asthma (Table 16). Previous guidelines (including the 1991, 1997, and 2002 NAEPP) had introduced asthma management strategies based solely on disease severity. The GINA guidelines also take the patient's response to therapy into account and accordingly create a classification based on how effectively the patient's asthma is controlled. The 2006 GINA report thus defines asthma control and bases treatment recommendations directly on its classification of three levels of control: controlled, partly controlled, and uncontrolled asthma (Table 15). GINA recommends that the previous asthma classification of intermittent; mild persistent; moderate persistent; and severe persistent not be entirely abandoned, and that it be used for research purposes rather than direct patient care.

GINA has pledged to update the Global Strategy for Asthma Management and Prevention on a regular basis.

Table 15   Asthma Treatment Goal: Control

Asthma is classified into three (3) categories, based on the level of control:

EPR-3 Guidelines Control Categories	GINA Guidelines Control Categories
Well-Controlled	Controlled
Not Well-Controlled	Partly Controlled
Very Poorly Controlled	Uncontrolled

Note: Although the EPR-3 & GINA guidelines use a different language to describe the three (3) categories of asthma control, they are conceptually concordant. More information about each is presented in Tables 25 and 26.

- The major goal of asthma treatment is the achievement and maintenance of clinical control.
- Ongoing asthma treatment is individualized and based on the degree of asthma control.
- Asthma therapy is organized around several "steps" that reflect the intensity of treatment required to obtain asthma control. A quick-relief, rapid-acting medicine is part of all steps, and controller medication is always required for steps 2–6.
- Asthma treatment is adjusted on a continual basis, based on the clinical response and the extent of asthma control. Medications should be stepped up promptly when control is lost and stepped down after control is achieved and maintained.
- Just as a person's asthma severity may vary over time, so too will the level of control, and thus the need for medication.
- The goal of asthma treatment = asthma control, in particular:
  - No (or rare) daytime asthma symptoms
  - No (or rare) nocturnal awakenings
  - No limitation of exercise
  - No limitation of daily, "routine" activities
  - Infrequent need for quick-relief, rapid-acting inhaled β_2 agonist bronchodilator for symptom relief ($\leq$ twice in any week)
  - Normal (or near normal) FEV_1 and/or PEF ($\geq$80% of predicted or of personal best values)
  - No exacerbations

The GINA experts have accordingly reviewed the impact of scientific asthma publications every 12 months and have published updates annually via the GINA Web site. The 2007 and 2008 updates to the 2006 Global

Table 16   GINA 2006 Classification and Guidelines: Main Points

Overall asthma severity is a function of both the severity of the underlying disease and its responsiveness to treatment.

Asthma is classified into one of three categories, based on the level of disease control:

- Controlled
- Partly Controlled
- Uncontrolled

The goal of asthma treatment is to achieve and maintain clinical control.

Treatment of an individual's asthma is based on their level of asthma control.

Treatment options are organized into five "steps" that reflect the intensity of treatment required to obtain asthma control. A reliever medication is part of all steps, and medications of the controller class are part of Steps 2–5.*

Asthma treatment should be adjusted on a continuously based level of asthma control: treatment should be stepped up when control is lost and brought back down when control is achieved.

The severity of a person's asthma may change over time, and the level of control may vary over time as well.

The goal of treatment and the definition of asthma control is:

- No more than twice a week for daytime symptoms
- No limitation of exercise, or of daily activities
- No nocturnal awakenings (or symptoms) because of asthma
- No more than twice a week need for reliever treatment
- Normal (or near-normal) lung function results
- No exacerbations or asthma "attacks"

*Note that the NAEPP differs slightly as it uses 6 steps of asthma treatment. Reliever medication is part of all steps, and medications of the controller class are part of Steps 2–6 in the NAEPP.

Strategy for Asthma Management and Prevention researched publications from July 1, 2006, to June 30, 2007, and from July 1, 2007, to June 30, 2008, respectively, and issued updates in December 2007 and again in 2008. The most recent edition continues to highlight the importance of asthma control and states.

there is now good evidence that the clinical manifestations of asthma, symptoms, sleep disturbances, limitations of daily activity, impairment of lung function, and use of rescue medications—can be controlled with appropriate treatment.

The ongoing NAEPP and GINA efforts to draft pragmatic guidelines and to revise them as our medical sophistication continues to grow ultimately benefits all persons with asthma. Physicians caring for persons with asthma (both children and adults) should be familiar with the documents. Information on where you can access and read the GINA guidelines if you are interested is included in Appendix 1.

35. What is cough-variant asthma?

Cough-variant asthma is a type of asthma in which cough is the dominant and sometimes only symptom. A person with cough-variant asthma experiences dry, generally nonproductive cough without wheezing or breathlessness (Table 17). The cough in that situation is considered to be a wheeze equivalent. The cough in cough-variant asthma may be provoked by triggers such as cold air or viral upper respiratory tract infections. Like "typical" asthma, there is usually a significant nocturnal component. Cough-variant asthma is more common in young children, yet has been described in all age groups, from toddlers to seniors. Since a chronic or longstanding cough can be a symptom of many different illnesses, confirming a diagnosis of cough-variant asthma may be challenging and requires a certain degree of suspicion from the onset. The chest X-ray is normal in cough-variant asthma, as are spirometry and other pulmonary-function tests. Evaluation may include undergoing bronchoprovocation testing, such as a methacholine challenge test. Some experts consider that a favorable

Viral

Caused by or related to a virus.

Cough-variant asthma is a type of asthma in which cough is the dominant and sometimes only symptom.

Table 17   Cough-Variant Asthma

Important points about cough-variant asthma include:

- Cough-variant asthma is a subclass, or variant, of asthma.
- Although individuals with asthma can experience cough as one symptom along with wheezing and breathlessness, individuals with the cough-variant form have only cough as a symptom, usually without wheezing or breathlessness.
- The chest X-ray is normal.
- Pulmonary function tests are normal.
- Methacholine challenge testing is abnormal, or "positive."
- Corticosteroids, either inhaled or in pill form, are effective treatments and should be part of the treatment regimen.
- The response to oral corticosteroids can be dramatic, with marked improvement in as little as 24 hours.
- A person with dry cough for three weeks or more should be evaluated for possible cough-variant asthma, especially if the chest X-ray and pulmonary function tests are normal.
- Other causes of chronic dry cough of three weeks' duration or more with normal chest X-ray and spirometry include: gastroesophageal reflux (GERD), postnasal drip or discharge, and cough following a viral respiratory illness.

Corticosteroids

Corticosteroids are hormones that are normally produced in very small quantities in health by the body's adrenal glands. Corticosteroids play a role in the regulation of blood pressure, as well as in the body's salt and water balance.

Oral

By mouth. Oral medications are taken by mouth and swallowed.

Antagonist

Something that opposes or resists the action of another. In medicine, an antagonist is a compound that prevents the effects or actions of a different compound.

response to a trial of appropriate asthma medicine clinches the diagnosis. Effective treatment typically requires anti-inflammatory corticosteroid medication. If there is no response to the inhaled form of corticosteroid after 8 weeks, then a course of oral (pill form) steroids is indicated, which can often yield prompt and dramatic improvement. Bronchodilators are often part of the treatment regimen, along with corticosteroids as cough-variant asthma does respond to standard therapies. Medication from the leukotriene antagonist class can also be effective. Studies indicate that up to 30% of individuals diagnosed with cough-variant asthma will, in time, go on to develop more typical asthma.

36. What is exercise-induced asthma (EIA)?

Exercise-induced asthma is an outdated phrase that makes little sense to an asthma specialist and that is confusing to boot! Exercise is a universal and common asthma trigger that is a cause of asthma symptoms when asthma is not optimally controlled. Any individual with inadequately controlled asthma will invariably experience variable cough, wheezing, and breathlessness with exertion and exercise. In the situation of poor asthma control, asthma symptoms are indeed exercise induced. In a subset of persons with asthma, however, exercise is the *only* precipitant of their asthma symptoms. Those persons have no symptoms of asthma and no decrease in lung function (peak flow or FEV_1) in the absence of exercise. The type of asthma arising *only* in the setting of exercise is classified as EIB for exercise-induced bronchoconstriction.

Individuals with EIB experience respiratory symptoms—most commonly a dry, nagging cough—in the setting of aerobic exercise. In addition to the cough, symptoms may include wheezing, shortness of breath, endurance problems, and chest discomfort such as tightness or painful sensations. The symptoms develop during (or minutes after) vigorous exercise and peak 5–10 minutes after cessation of the activity. EIB lessens thereafter and abates 30–45 minutes later. Since symptoms and lung function findings tests are only present with exercise, confirming the diagnosis can be tricky! Many persons initially thought to have EIB actually have a diagnosis of usual asthma that needs to become better controlled; symptoms of their underlying asthma become triggered by exercise. The treating physician should suspect EIB when there is a pattern of asthma symptoms and lung function abnormality only during and immediately following exertion. An exercise-challenge test may be helpful in establishing the diagnosis.

Treatment of EIB includes proper attention to warm-up and cool-down maneuvers, as well as prescription medication. Medicines effective in the treatment of

EIB include oral leukotriene modifiers and anti-inflammatory medicines, as well as inhalers such as inhaled short-acting β_2 agonists, and/or inhaled cromolyn or nedocromil. When inhalers are prescribed, they should be used about 20 minutes prior to the warm-up routine as a preventive measure. Inhalers may otherwise be required after exercise to accelerate resolution of symptoms. It is important to treat EIB in order to allow for full, symptom-free participation in sports, fitness, and recreational activities that are part of a healthy lifestyle. Many world-class athletes carry a diagnosis of EIB, proving that asthma is not a barrier to athletic achievement. Parents should notify teachers and coaches that a student has EIB; the youngster should take prescribed medication before sports and should take part in athletics and all physical education offerings. A competitive athlete with EIB must disclose asthma medication use and should become familiar with the U.S. Anti-Doping Agency requirements, which are available at http://www.usantidoping.org. As of this writing and subject to change, use of some inhaled bronchodilator asthma medications (salmeterol, formoterol, salbutamol, terbutaline) requires that the athlete complete a therapeutic use exemption (TUE) form. Additionally, inhaled corticosteroid medication must be declared, and prescription of corticosteroid medication in pill (oral) form requires a TUE form.

In EIB, airway narrowing (bronchoconstriction) occurs secondary to vigorous exercise. The mechanism responsible for EIB implicates inhalation of cool dry air, specifically, fluxes in humidity and temperature within the airways during rapid breathing. EIB occurs more commonly with certain types of exercise, such as long-distance running. Competitive sports that require prolonged periods of strenuous activity, such as soccer, tennis, distance cycling, Nordic skiing, and cross-country running, will more often trigger EIB symptoms than activities such as baseball or swimming. EIB can occur in any weather, yet is more likely in cool and dry environments than in warmer, more humid ones. Up to one quarter of Olympic winter sports athletes experience EIB, with the highest numbers (50%) in cross-country skiers. In contrast, the U.S. Olympic Committee determined that 11.2% of athletes competing in the 1984 Summer Olympics experienced EIB. Although EIB requires treatment, it does not reflect inadequately controlled underlying asthma. Some physicians consider it a subtype of asthma while others view it as a possible precursor to asthma and continue to monitor their patients with EIB for the emergence of more usual forms of asthma as time goes by.

Gemma's comment:

My daughter was not diagnosed with asthma until she was in her 20s, but she now feels that she had EIB as a teenager when she began running with school teams. Outdoors, and especially in cold weather, she would have trouble breathing while exercising, but when she stopped she would recover quickly and feel that the problem had gone away. She was, and is, very athletic, and particularly devoted to running. At the time, she didn't complain of breathing problems and no coach ever noticed them. I should add that she is still an avid runner, but now she carries a bronchodilator with her and is careful about running in very cold weather or when the air seems especially polluted.

37. What is the asthmatic triad?

The first report of what is now called the asthmatic triad appeared in 1922 in *La Presse Médicale,* a French medical journal. The authors of the report, Widal, Abrami, and Lermoyez, described an association between sensitivity to aspirin—introduced commercially by the Bayer Company by 1899—and the occurrence of nasal polyps and asthma. In the late 1960s, Dr. Max Samter published a series of articles characterizing the triad and further elucidated the nature of the aspirin intolerance. Dr. Samter greatly advanced knowledge in the area, and in recognition of the fact, the asthmatic triad is also known as Samter's syndrome.

Aspirin, or acetylsalicylic acid, is a widely prescribed and consumed drug with beneficial anti-inflammatory, anti-fever, and pain-relieving properties. It is also useful for its blood thinning effects in the treatment of heart diseases and in certain types of stroke prevention. The consumption of aspirin in the United States has been estimated at approximately 80 billion tablets per year. In many ways, aspirin is an ideal medication: inexpensive, safe, and highly effective. In some people with asthma, however, aspirin carries a real risk. The term *aspirin-induced asthma*, or *AIA*, refers to the development of wheezing and bronchoconstriction after the ingestion of aspirin, or aspirin-like products called NSAIDs—non-steroidal anti-inflammatory drugs. AIA usually occurs in the setting of severe, chronic asthma and is more common among females. Approximately 10–20% of people with asthma also have AIA. The NAEPP reports that 21% of all adults with asthma and 5% of children with asthma have AIA. It is estimated that, of those asthmatics with AIA, 50% have steroid-dependent asthma classified as severe persistent, 30% have moderate persistent disease, and 20% have mild persistent or intermittent asthma.

Symptoms of AIA include, first and foremost, an acute exacerbation of asthma within 3 hours of taking aspirin or one of the NSAIDs. Respiratory symptoms include wheezing, cough, and breathlessness, secondary to bronchoconstriction and inflammation. The acute chest

Non-steroidal anti-inflammatory drugs (NSAIDs)

Potent anti-inflammatory drugs, widely prescribed for the treatment of pain, fever, and conditions such as arthritis. Some NSAIDs are available over the counter; others require a physician's prescription.

Acute

Short-lived, brief, sudden, not drawn out. Chronic is the opposite of acute. A virus such as influenza will cause an acute illness that may last a few weeks.

symptoms are accompanied by nasal, eye, and skin symptoms including severe runny nose; red, puffy, itchy eyes; and flushing and reddening of the skin of the face or neck. The asthmatic exacerbation can be quite severe and may require emergency room treatment or even admission to hospital. AIA is a cause of near-fatal asthma. Studies have suggested that up to 25% of all persons with asthma admitted to hospital in respiratory failure requiring intensive care and ventilator support may have had the event precipitated by aspirin or NSAID ingestion.

Treatment of AIA consists of lifelong aspirin and NSAID avoidance (Tables 18 and 19). The oral leukotriene

Table 18   Medicines to Avoid in Aspirin-Induced Asthma

Aspirin or acetylsalicylic acid

"Pure" aspirin is available over the counter without a prescription, in generic and non-generic (or brand) formulations. Examples include: acetylsalicylic acid (generic), Ascriptin, Bayer, Bufferin, Ecotrin, Empirin, Halfprin, and St. Joseph. Look at the list of ingredients carefully for the words *aspirin* or *acetylsalicylic acid*, alone or in combination.

Aspirin-containing formulations

Many remedies contain aspirin as an ingredient, combined with other medicines. These remedies include both over-the-counter and prescription formulations. In the first category are products such as: Alka Seltzer Plus, Anacin, Aspergum, Doan's Pills, Excedrin, Goody's Headache Powders, Pamprin, Pepto Bismol products, and others. Many products you see on the shelves in addition to those listed here may contain aspirin. They may be labeled for treatment of arthritis pain, cold symptoms, headache, indigestion, menstrual pain, pain from minor sprains or injury, and sinus symptoms. Make sure to check the list of ingredients carefully and look for the words *aspirin* or *acetylsalicylic acid*, alone or in combination.

Prescription medicines that contain aspirin are also very common, and are often used for pain control and relief. Some such medicines are Darvon, Fiorinal, Percodan, Talwin, and Zorprin. Make certain that all your treating doctors know that you have AIA, and that you must avoid taking aspirin, as well as NSAIDs. Check to make sure that the pharmacist who fills your prescription is aware of your aspirin sensitivity. Read any inserts provided with the prescribed medicine.

NSAIDs

NSAIDs include a large number of products, including both over-the-counter and prescription drugs. NSAIDs are useful in pain and arthritis treatment. Some of the most commonly used NSAIDs are ibuprofen (Advil, Motrin) and naprosyn (Aleve), which are available without a prescription. Newer Cox-2 medications such as celecoxib (Celebrex) and valdecoxib (Bextra) should likewise be avoided.

Table 19   "Safe" Medicines in Aspirin-Induced Asthma

- Your physician and your pharmacist are professionals who can provide you with information about the safety of both prescription and over-the-counter medications in AIA. You have a responsibility to inform them that you have a diagnosis of AIA and should ask them any questions you have about any medicine.

- Many of the products you must avoid are used in the treatment of pain (headache, menstrual cramps, sprains, and injuries) and inflammatory conditions (arthritis, osteoarthritis). A list of the generic name of medicines that are usually considered safe by medical experts follows:

  - Acetaminophen
  - Sodium salicylate
  - Salicylamide
  - Choline magnesium trisalicylate
  - Benzydamine
  - Chloroquine
  - Azapropazone
  - Dextropropoxyphene

Aspirin desensitization is a special, individualized treatment that eventually permits an individual with AIA to tolerate regular, daily doses of aspirin.

Desensitization

Reduction or elimination of an allergic sensitivity or reaction to a specific allergen. Immunotherapy (allergy shots) is generally used to achieve desensitization in patients with allergies.

modifier medications (zafirlukast, zileuton, and montelukast) are useful in blocking and preventing the response to aspirin and NSAIDs to a variable extent in AIA. If aspirin therapy is deemed essential for medical reasons, then the person with asthma and AIA should be referred to an allergist with expertise in aspirin desensitization. Aspirin desensitization is a special, individualized treatment that eventually permits an individual with AIA to tolerate regular, daily doses of aspirin. Desensitization could, for example, be considered in the case of a man with aspirin-induced asthma who is recuperating from a heart attack and whose cardiologist believes that a small daily dose of aspirin is essential in preventing a second heart attack.

38. What is occupational asthma?

Gemma's comment:

I worked for many years in a large public building, which was often described as a "sick" building, in part because of its faulty ventilating system. I often noticed breathing problems, especially when water in the radiators leaked, leaving the industrial carpeting on my office floor damp and probably moldy. Although the building was studied several times by environmentalist specialists and always found to be sick, public funds to fix these problems were never made available.

Occupational asthma describes asthma that is caused by exposure to a precise, defined substance in the workplace environment. Although figures vary from country to country and are difficult to pinpoint, it is estimated that 5–15% of newly diagnosed asthma in working adults is due to occupational (or workplace) exposure. Many physicians fail to consider the possibility of occupational asthma in adults with newly identified asthma and can remain unaware of the disease specifics. Symptoms of occupational asthma may be indistinguishable from those of classic asthma. An astute physician will inquire about current and past jobs held by an adult in whom asthma is newly diagnosed. Another clue to the diagnosis can be provided by close observation of any temporal associations between work, leisure time, and respiratory symptoms. The NAEPP's *Expert Panel Report-3* points out "occupational asthma is suggested by a correlation between asthma symptoms and work, as well as with improvement when away from work for several days." Serial peak flow measurements during an entire month, for example, while at work as well as on weekends or days off, can be helpful in identifying patterns that might suggest occupational asthma. It is crucial to recognize occupational

An astute physician will inquire about current and past jobs held by an adult in whom asthma is newly diagnosed.

asthma because the key to successful treatment is prompt removal of the patient from the workplace exposure that is causing the asthma. If occupational asthma is properly identified in a timely manner, and if the exposure to the offending agent ceases within a certain period of time, then the prognosis is favorable. If exposure continues, however, there is a "point of no return" past which a person with occupational asthma may have permanent respiratory symptoms and disability, even if the exposure ceases at a later date.

Occupational asthma is different from work-aggravated asthma. Work-aggravated asthma refers to preexisting asthma that worsens at work. For example, a person with a history of easily controlled asthma in adolescence might develop an increase in asthma symptoms as an adult when working outdoors during cold winter months. Another example of work-aggravated asthma involves asthma that worsens at work because of irritant exposures, such as might be the case for a bartender with asthma working in a restaurant full of cigarette smoke or an indoor parking garage attendant whose asthma flares from inhaling automobile exhaust fumes.

True occupational, or work-related, asthma is a potentially serious medical condition with significant socioeconomic repercussions. The immunologist and allergist Dr. David I. Bernstein's 1993 characterization of occupational asthma has been widely accepted as the standard definition of the disease. The definition states,

Occupational asthma is a disease characterized by variable air flow limitation and/or airway hyper-responsiveness due to causes and conditions attributable to a particular occupational environment and not to stimuli encountered outside the workplace.

Immunologist

A specialist in the science of immunology, which is concerned with various phenomena of immunity, sensitivity, and allergy.

There are two general types of true occupational asthma (OA). Experts have classified the two types as asthma with latency and asthma without latency. The first type of OA is asthma that develops over time, caused by repeated inhalation of sensitizing work exposures to a specific substance, usually a large protein. Examples of sensitizing agents include formaldehyde, mineral dusts, animal proteins, flours, and grains. More than 250 different workplace substances have been reported to cause occupational asthma. Different manufacturing industries are involved, from baking, to veterinary work, to paint and circuit board production. Interestingly, not all workers in a certain industry and with clear-cut exposure actually go on to develop asthma. Studies suggest that atopy and cigarette smoking may predispose some persons to the development of occupational asthma. The second, more unusual type of OA involves the emergence of new asthma after a single, intense, and often dramatic exposure to potent respiratory irritants, such as bleach, chlorine gas, or strong acids, for example. Chemical spills and workplace accidents are often implicated. The term *RADS* describes reactive airways dysfunction syndrome, a type of OA without latency that begins abruptly, usually within 24 hours of an intense, inhaled-irritant exposure that persists for longer than 3 months and behaves like typical asthma.

Occupational asthma is more than a single entity, as this answer clearly indicates. If OA is suspected, medical evaluation and consultation by an occupational health physician should be considered.

Atopy

An inherited predisposition to the development of allergic conditions such as hay fever, eczema, allergic rhinitis, and even certain forms of asthma. A person with evidence of atopy is said to be atopic.

39. What is an asthma action plan?

The National Asthma Education and Prevention Program's *EPR-3* emphasizes patient education and the forging of an ongoing active partnership between the patient and the treating healthcare provider in order to ensure optimal asthma treatment. The clinician has, without question, a continuing responsibility to educate every patient about their own asthma and to teach what constitutes good asthma control, how to identify and treat flares of asthma symptoms, how prescribed asthma medication works, and what doses are indicated. Understanding so much information may seem daunting at first, but it need not be. Learning self-management of asthma is a feature of effective asthma care and leads to improved outcomes. An asthma action plan is a component of the ongoing teaching and information exchange between patients and the healthcare team. It consists of a written and personalized set of instructions for self-monitoring and asthma management. The most recent *EPR-3* asthma guidelines advise that clinicians "provide all patients with a written asthma action plan that includes two aspects: (1) daily management and (2) how to recognize and handle worsening asthma." The action plan should ideally be crafted at the time of the patient's first visit and should be subject to review and revisions at follow-up visits. The written plan emphasizes asthma control, regular use of maintenance medications, patient observations and self-monitoring, and provides written guidelines for treatment of increasing symptomatology and exacerbated asthma (Table 20). Previous asthma treatment guidelines, such as the 1997 and 2002 NAEPP reports, advocated that each patient be provided two documents, both a written individualized daily self-management plan, and an asthma action plan. The practical, real-life use of two plans quickly became confusing and cumbersome all around. The 2007 *EPR-3* guidelines recognize "confusion over the previous guidelines' use of different terms" and advocates for a single written asthma action plan.

Learning self-management of asthma is a feature of effective asthma care and leads to improved outcomes.

Table 20   Asthma Action Plans

Asthma action plans may be based on symptoms, PEF measurements, or both, depending on the patient's preference as well as that of the healthcare provider.

Asthma action plans should always be provided **in writing** in the context of an ongoing partnership between the patient with asthma and the healthcare provider.

Asthma action plans should be subject to ongoing review and adjustment during follow-up asthma visits.

Asthma action plans are recommended for patients who have:

• moderate persistent asthma
• severe persistent asthma
• a history of severe exacerbations
• poorly controlled asthma of any severity

An asthma action plan MUST include clear instructions for:

• **daily asthma management**: what medicines to take, with names and dosages, environmental control measures
• **recognizing worsening asthma**: what signs, symptoms to look for, measure PEF
• **handling worsening asthma**: what medicines to take, with names and dosages, when to go to an ER, when to call 911
• **proper adjustment of medication dosing**

See a sample Asthma Action Plan at: http://www.cdc.gov/ASTHMA/ actionplan.html

The key feature of any written asthma plan is that it is individualized. Just as two people with asthma will have different manifestations of their disease, so, too, will they have different treatments and different action plans. A person whose intermittent asthma typically exacerbates when he is suffering from a chest cold, for example, will likely have instructions in his plan to begin taking inhaled steroid medication if he notices exertional breathlessness and a drop in his PEF values. Another person, whose asthma symptoms are triggered by late summer ragweed allergy, will perhaps have to restart her leukotriene receptor antagonist medication and her prescribed inhaled medicines when she notes increased cough as ragweed counts rise. Another point to remember is that if you have been provided with an action plan, it should be reviewed and revised (as needed) at every visit. Sample asthma plans can be found on the Internet. Simply use your favorite browser and type "written asthma action plan" in the search window. Alternatively, you can review a sample asthma action plan on the CDC Web site at www.cdc.gov/asthma/actionplan.html.

Despite the strong recommendations of the NAEPP, as well as enthusiastic support from professional medical societies and managed care insurance companies, written asthma plans are not universally popular in the asthma community. Polls show most asthma patients prefer having a written plan of action. Many doctors, however, especially physicians practicing in private practice rather than in clinic or hospital settings, dislike written asthma plans. The most common reason for a person with asthma not following a written action plan is quite simply that his or her physician has never provided one! Written action plans are particularly recommended for persons (of any age) whose asthma is classified as either moderate persistent or severe persistent, who have a history of severe exacerbations, or whose asthma is poorly controlled.

Studies of written action plans, both in the United States and abroad, have yielded inconsistent results; nevertheless, the consensus of several recently published studies is that implementation of an asthma action plan leads to fewer emergency room visits and lower asthma hospitalization rates. Most patients, especially children, clearly benefit from written asthma plans. Other studies suggest that it is not the written plan itself that improves outcomes, but rather the effects of the focused attention of the physician, self-management asthma education and teaching, and the enhanced interaction between patient and healthcare provider. In other words, as long as the proper information on recognizing symptoms, tuning in to loss of asthma control, and appropriate medication adjustment is provided and understood, the outcome is improved regardless of whether instructions are given in writing as part of a plan or verbally during an office visit or in a telephone conversation.

40. Why should I take asthma medicine if I feel fine?

Perhaps the biggest asthma myth circulating today is summed up in the phrase *no symptoms means no asthma.* Wrong! The correct concept is "no symptoms means I still have asthma; I feel fine because my asthma is well controlled." Two distinct clinical scenarios apply when asthma symptoms become imperceptible and you feel fine. Either your asthma is on the milder part of the asthma severity spectrum, intermittent (based on the NAEPP classification) in nature, and in remission, or it is one of the more persistent types of asthma and your taking your anti-asthma medication is keeping it under good control. Asthma medicine can be classified into two broad categories: as-needed, rapid-acting, quick-relief treatments, and long-term, maintenance control, daily-use treatments (see Question 54). Adults and children with intermittent asthma take their medicine only when they are actively symptomatic. They do not require any preprogrammed daily medicine. Others with more pronounced asthma, classified as persistent, must take maintenance controller medicine every day even though they may become free of symptoms and feel perfectly well.

A major advance in the medical profession's understanding of asthma is the recognition of the crucial role of lung and airway inflammation. If an individual with asthma has ongoing lung inflammation, his or her asthma is not effectively controlled, and that in turn leads to the individual experiencing one or more asthma symptoms. Too many people with inadequately treated asthma "adapt" to abnormal lung function and, consciously or not, learn to "live" with their symptoms. I clearly recall, for example, a middle-aged patient of mine who during her initial visit with me reported that she would always take a taxi to and from work in Manhattan all winter long despite the expense. Rather than walk, wait for a bus, or take the subway, she always preferred to go by cab during the winter because of the development of cold-induced dry cough and uncomfortable breathing. When the temperature would dip below 40°F, she could walk only very brief distances before she would experience cough and breathlessness. She was, when I first met her, proud of how she had "learned to live with asthma," which she referred to as her "condition." She believed then that she was a model patient by toughing it out. She was mistaken in her assumption that she needed to make accommodations for her asthma, and did not realize that she should instead have been taking a combination of asthma medicine, which would have allowed her to become free of asthma symptoms despite still having asthma.

In asthma management, a primary treatment goal is the absence of daily daytime and nighttime symptoms. Your breathing should be comfortable all the time. During a normal day, you should have no awareness of your breathing, which should be quiet, effortless, and automatic. If your asthma falls into a classification other than the NAEPP's intermittent, then you are likely to be prescribed daily controller medication along with quick-relief inhaled medicine as I did for my taxi-traveler patient. The controller medicine addresses the inflammatory component of asthma. The medicine is designed to be taken daily, around the clock, to keep the inflammation controlled and quiescent. It is a preventive medicine. You should use it as prescribed, *especially* if you have no symptoms. The fact that you have no symptoms means that the medicine is working perfectly! Continue taking it! If you stop your medicine because you feel fine, you may not feel fine for long. Rather than stop your medicine on your own, contact your asthma doctor to review the circumstances. The fact that you feel healthy certainly indicates that your treatment has been effective. It may also be a hint that now that your asthma symptoms have responded to treatment, you may be ready to step down or decrease the amount of medicine you are using for asthma control. Experts advise that, as a rule, asthma be well controlled for 3 months (90 consecutive days) and that lung function tests be within a normal (or close to normal) range before proceeding with a step down in asthma medication.

What happened to my patient who suffered daily symptoms from Thanksgiving until Easter? After her first visit several years ago, and the prescription of two different inhalers, she was no longer symptomatic in the cold weather. Together we learned that her asthma requires only infrequent doses of inhaled, short-acting β_2 agonist (quick-relief) bronchodilator therapy in the spring and summer for control. In the late fall and through the winter, she needs to take additional medicine daily. She begins using the additional controller inhalers as soon as

If you stop your medicine because you feel fine, you may not feel fine for long.

Experts advise that, as a rule, asthma be well controlled for 3 months (90 consecutive days) and that lung function tests be within a normal (or close to normal) range before proceeding with a step down in asthma medication.

Asthma: Classification and Variants

93

the weather cools and before she develops the cold air-induced cough and breathlessness. Now that she has control over her asthma, she has more choices of how to get to work! She also decided to get a small dog (which she had always wanted) and proudly walks the pup before and after work, in all kinds of nasty weather!

PART FOUR

Asthma: Treatment Plans, Goals, and Strategies

What are asthma triggers?

What are the goals of asthma treatment?

What makes a doctor an asthma specialist and how can I find out if my physician is a specialist in asthma care?

Do I need to consult a physician who specializes in asthma?

My asthma is active; how do I know whether I should go to the nearest hospital emergency room?

More . . .

41. What are asthma triggers?

Gemma's comment:

My daughter and I seem to be especially sensitive to certain foods, like soy and nuts. My daughter feels that if she has a cold, the skin of some foods (e.g., peaches and eggplant) makes her throat close up. I, too, have had such symptoms, but I think that food sensitivities, which are quite different from taste preferences, change over time.

Asthma triggers are exposures that precipitate or worsen a person's asthma.

Asthma triggers are exposures that precipitate or worsen a person's asthma (Table 21). Some triggers are considered universal. Most people with asthma will notice that a viral respiratory infection, bronchitis, or a chest cold will increase asthma symptoms. Inhalation of cold air and strenuous aerobic exercise are also common triggers.

Table 21   Asthma Triggers

Asthma triggers are exposures that precipitate or worsen a person's asthma. A person with asthma may have more than one trigger. Some triggers are nearly universal among persons with asthma; others are more individual.

- Allergens
  Common examples include pets (such as cats or dogs), foods (such as peanuts, tree nuts, shellfish), or aeroallergens (such as ragweed, grasses, or pollens)
- Cold air
- Cigarette smoke
- Exercise
- Infections: viral or bacterial
  - Bronchitis/chest colds
  - Pneumonia
  - Sinusitis
- Irritants
- Medications
- Stress
- Sulfites

By correctly identifying your asthma triggers and avoiding exposure to those triggers, your asthma will be better controlled.

Table 22   Key Components of Effective Asthma Management

Identification of factors ("triggers") that worsen your asthma

Avoidance of factors ("triggers") that worsen your asthma

Taking appropriate **medication** for your asthma

• Daily controller medication(s)

• Quick-relief medication(s)

Monitoring your asthma to assess for degree of **control**

Following your **asthma action plan**

Other triggers are more individual or idiosyncratic. Strong odors or perfumes, as well as cigarette smoke, can all be asthma triggers. Persons with asthma who also have specific allergies will notice that allergens can be asthma triggers. This is often the case in a cat-allergic person, for example, who begins to experience chest discomfort, tightness, wheezing, and shortness of breath after visiting a home with cats in residence. Some foods, sulfite food additives, as well as certain medications can trigger asthmatic symptoms in susceptible persons. The importance of identifying an individual's asthma triggers cannot be overstated as exposure to triggers often underlies asthma exacerbations and can lead to loss of asthma control. Modern asthma treatment includes identification of each patient's asthma triggers in order to avoid exposure to them as much as possible (Table 22). By completely avoiding, or at least minimizing, exposure to triggers, asthma symptoms are greatly reduced. If avoidance of known triggers is effective, asthma medication can often be decreased (stepped down) as asthma symptoms come under long-term control.

Kerrin's comment:

It wasn't difficult to figure out that every time my son got a cold, his asthma symptoms would flare. The doctor gave us our nebulizer the first time our son got a bad cold because he was

Modern asthma treatment includes identification of each patient's asthma triggers in order to avoid exposure to them as much as possible.

wheezing. The second time he got a bad cold, he ended up in the hospital for breathing treatments every 2 hours and had to stay in an oxygen tent. Now whenever he starts to sneeze continually and we see his nose starting to run, we get the nebulizer out and start giving him preventive treatments to try to stave off the worst. We also figured out quickly that another trigger for my son's asthma was exposure to dogs. His second trip to the emergency room, which led to another overnight stay in the hospital, occurred after visiting my mother's house where two dogs live (even though they are supposed to be hypoallergenic dogs, which I was later told by my son's pediatric allergy specialist is impossible no matter what the breed). We haven't been back to my mother's house for well over a year and a half.

42. What are the goals of asthma treatment?

The fundamental goal of asthma therapy is the control of all symptoms, which in turn leads to normalization of lung function and prevention of exacerbations and hospitalizations and allows for an active, healthy lifestyle (Table 23). Once control is established, ongoing, successful treatment may include daily prescription medication, such as inhaled bronchodilators and anti-inflammatory medicines, a regular exercise regimen, and environmental control measures (Table 24).

Table 23   Elements of Asthma Control: What to Look For

Monitor SYMPTOM frequency—keep an eye on each of four key indicators and their frequency:

- Daytime symptoms
- Exercise limitation
- Limitation of daily activities
- Nocturnal (nighttime) awakenings

Observe MEDICINE use—how many times a week quick-relief, rapid-acting inhaled β_2 agonist bronchodilator is required for symptom relief.

Check LUNG FUNCTION TESTS—pulmonary function tests include the FEV_1 test and peak flow measurements (PEF).

Follow EXACERBATION frequency—how many exacerbations occur.

Table 24   Asthma Treatment

- Patient education: asthma physiology, proper use of medicines, self-monitoring, asthma action plans
- Pharmacological treatment: when and how to use medicines
- Environmental controls and modifications: identify allergens and minimize or eliminate exposure, especially in the home and in the patient's bedroom
- Trigger identification and avoidance
- Alliance between patient and caregiver
- Treatment includes an emphasis and focus on preventive therapy, not merely on symptomatic therapy

Physicians and their patients should work together to attain an asymptomatic state, free of bothersome breathing symptoms such as cough, breathlessness, or nighttime awakenings. Such collaboration requires attention and interest from both partners, with a constructive and clear dialogue and a commitment to the goal at hand. It may take several visits to learn about your asthma and to understand how the medicines work and how to take them. Asthma is a condition that requires a commitment and work on the part of the patient in order to achieve treatment goals. Learning the correct technique of inhaling asthma medicine from a metered-dose inhaler (MDI) or dry-powder inhaler (DPI), for example, may be frustrating at first and may require time and patience. Questions 62 and 63 review how best to use inhalers. If you are not certain that you understand how to inhale your medicine, or you are not sure you know what your doctor is talking about, speak up! Make certain you report symptoms you are experiencing. Your doctor should want to know of any new or worsening asthma symptoms; don't be concerned about "upsetting" the doctor.

Adherence to the medicine prescribed for asthma treatment is crucial for successful asthma treatment, which is why I advocate that each person with asthma learn

Asymptomatic

Without any manifestations or symptoms of disease or illness. The major goal of asthma treatment is to achieve an asymptomatic state so that the person with asthma experiences no symptoms whatsoever and is able to lead a full and productive life.

Asthma is a condition that requires a commitment and work on the part of the patient in order to achieve treatment goals.

about the medicine they take, how it works to help asthma, and how often it should be taken. An effective asthma regimen will succeed in achieving a minimal requirement for short-acting β_2 agonist quick-relief medication. It will also ensure minimal, if any, medication side effects. Lung function should normalize with proper asthma care, and monitoring of the FEV_1 can and should be performed in children as well as teens and adults. All asthma symptoms should be absent or minimal during the daytime as well as at night. Sleep should be restful and uninterrupted. There should be no absences from work or school due to asthma. Exacerbations should also be few (or none) and far between (Tables 25 and 26). If an exacerbation does

Table 25   Assessing Your Asthma Control: GINA

Characteristic	Controlled Asthma	Partly Controlled Asthma	Uncontrolled Asthma
Daytime symptoms	No more often than twice in one week	More often than twice a week	If three (or more) characteristics of asthma are partly controlled during a one-week period, the asthma becomes classified as uncontrolled
Activity limitation	None	Any	
Night-time symptoms	None	Any	
Need for quick-relief, rapid-acting inhaled β_2 agonist bronchodilator	No more often than twice a week for symptom relief	More often than twice a week for symptom relief	
Lung function tests*: FEV_1 or PEF	Normal range FEV_1 PEF > 80% personal best	FEV_1 less than 80% of predicted PEF less than 80% of personal best	
Exacerbations	None in the last year	One or more in a year	One in any week**

Notes:

*Lung function tests are not considered reliable in children younger than 5 years of age, so this characteristic applies only to older children, teenagers, and adults.

**An exacerbation during a week makes that week an "uncontrolled" asthma week.

Source: Adapted from the 2008 GINA report.

Asthma: Treatment Plans, Goals, and Strategies

Table 26   Assessing Asthma Control in Older Children and in Adults: NAEPP

Components of Asthma Control	Asthma Control in Persons aged 12 years and older		
	Well-Controlled Asthma	Not Well-Controlled	Very Poorly Controlled
Symptoms	< 2 days/week	> 2 days/week	All day
Night-time awakenings	< 2 × a month	1–3 × a week	≥ 4 × a week
Interference with normal activities	No limitation	No limitation	Very limited activities
Use of quick-relief, rapid-acting inhaled β_2 agonist bronchodilator for symptom relief	< 2 days/week	> 2 days/week	Several times a day
FEV_1 or Peak Expiratory Flow (PEF)	> 80% predicted > 80% personal best	60–80% predicted/personal best	< 60% predicted < 60% personal best
Exacerbations*	0 to 1 per year	> 2 per year	

*Comment: The NAEPP's *EPR-3* states that in general, more frequent and intense exacerbations (e.g., requiring urgent, unscheduled care, hospitalization, or ICU admission) indicate poorer disease control. For treatment purposes, patients who had ≥ 2 exacerbations requiring oral systemic corticosteroids may be considered the same as patients who have asthma that is not well-controlled, even in the absence of impairment levels consistent with not-well-controlled asthma.

Source: Modified and adapted from the 2007 NAEPP's *EPR-3*.

develop, it should be recognized immediately and treated aggressively. When people can forget that they have asthma, except for the fact that they have to take medicine, and when they can fully participate in work, play, and sports, and enjoy life without limitation, then the principal goal of asthma treatment has been met.

43. Will asthma lead to loss of oxygen?

Well-controlled, stable, treated asthma does not affect the lungs' ability to extract needed oxygen from the air we breathe. Severe exacerbations of asthma, however, have the potential to significantly interfere with the lungs' capacity to obtain oxygen from the air around us and send it into the body. When ongoing inflammation, bronchospasm, and mucus accumulation narrow the bronchial passages, oxygen levels may decrease. The emergency treatment of an asthma exacerbation that brings a patient to the emergency room, for example, always begins with supplemental oxygen, given by an oxygen mask or by nasal prongs. In an asthma emergency, it is always better to err on the side of safety and automatically prescribe supplemental oxygen, rather than risk reduced oxygen. Once an asthma exacerbation resolves and control of asthma is regained, oxygen levels return to normal; thankfully no permanent or long-term change affects oxygenation!

A pulse oximeter is a small portable device that provides a noninvasive way of determining if the body's oxygen levels are normal or reduced. A pulse oximeter measures oxygen percent saturation through a painless sensor that is usually placed on a fingertip covering the nail bed. Pulse oximetry can be performed any place healthcare is provided—in a clinic, doctor's office, ambulance, emergency room, or hospital. It is also standard practice to monitor patients undergoing anesthesia with continuous pulse oximeter measurements. I am often asked what a normal reading is, and as a rule, a value of 95% or more indicates adequate oxygen levels. A healthy person with well-controlled asthma can be expected to have oximetry readings of 95–100%. Variations can be due to nonpulmonary factors, such as age, altitude, and degree of fitness. Other ways doctors assess oxygenation is by physical examination (a blue discoloration of the lips or of the nail beds, called cyanosis, indicates inadequate oxygen) and by direct sampling of blood from an artery—an arterial blood gas, or ABG, as explained in Question 30.

Bronchospasm

Abnormal contraction of the bronchial smooth muscles.

Cyanosis

An abnormal physical examination finding that correlates with abnormally low levels of blood oxygen. Cyanosis is a bluish discoloration best detected in the nail beds (under the fingernails) and around the lips.

44. What makes a doctor an asthma specialist and how can I find out if my physician is a specialist in asthma care?

An asthma specialist is a physician who has a special interest in treating patients with asthma and who has completed postdoctoral training either in adult or pediatric lung diseases (pulmonary medicine) or in allergy and immunology (Table 27). A physician is a medical doctor who has graduated first from college and then from medical school. After medical school, a future asthma specialist will continue postdoctoral training, previously termed *internship* and *residency*, for 3–4 years in a broad field such as adult internal medicine, family practice, or pediatrics. Much of this time is spent in a hospital setting or in a clinic. After internship and residency training, the future asthma specialist will spend an additional 3–5 years in even more specialized training. Such additional training is called a fellowship. Fellowships in the fields of adult pulmonary medicine lead to adult asthma specialization, whereas those in the field of pediatric pulmonology train asthma specialists for children. Fellowships in allergy and immunology train physicians to care for asthma patients of all ages.

There are two types of medical schools in the United States. The majority of accredited American medical schools, numbering 131 as of this writing, are allopathic medical schools and grant the M.D. degree after 4 years of postcollege study. Five states do not have a medical school: Alaska, Delaware, Idaho, Montana, and Wyoming. There are also currently 25 American colleges of osteopathic medicine, offering instruction at 31 locations in 22 states with far fewer students enrolled than in allopathic medical schools. Osteopathic schools grant the D.O. degree. The D.O. stands for doctor of

Allopath

A physician graduate of an allopathic medical school. The majority of medical schools in the United States are allopathic and confer the MD degree. The original meaning of allopath is that of a physician trained in (or who practices) allopathy. Allopathy historically involved treating diseases with remedies that produced effects different from those produced by the disease itself.

Osteopath

A practitioner of osteopathy, a school of medicine originally based upon the concept that the body in correct alignment becomes efficient at making its own remedies against illness. Osteopaths today are physician graduates of osteopathic medical schools.

Table 27 Physicians' Qualifications and Specialties

MD	Your physician is an allopathic medical school graduate.
DO	Your physician is an osteopathic medical school graduate.
"Board Certified" The American Board of Medical Specialties includes: ABAI—American Board of Allergy & Immunology (www.abai.org) ABIM—American Board of Internal Medicine* (www.abim.org) ABPed—American Board of Pediatrics (www.abp.org) *You can check to see that your asthma physician is board certified by the ABIM on the Internet. Go to: www.abim.org/services/verify-a-physician.aspx	The American Board of Medical Specialties (www.abms.org) sanctions 24 medical specialties. Each different medical Board evaluates M.D. and D.O. candidates who voluntarily present for evaluation of their credentials and qualifications. The qualified candidate physician then takes a specialized examination. The successful candidate is then certified by the specific Board. Most Boards require recertification at specific time intervals.
FACP	Your physician is a Fellow of the American College of Physicians, a mark of distinction for an internist or physician specialized in the medical care of adults. The ACP (www.acponline.org) is a professional society.
FAAP	Your physician is a Fellow of the American Academy of Pediatrics, a mark of distinction for a pediatrician or physician specialized in the medical care of children and adolescents. The AAP (www.aap.org) is a professional society.
FAAFP	Your physician is a Fellow of the American Academy of Family Physicians, a mark of distinction for a family practitioner or physician specialized in the general care of persons from infancy onward through adulthood. The AAFP (www.aafp.org) is a professional society.
FCCP	Your physician is a Fellow of the American College of Chest Physicians, a professional society dedicated to the treatment of lung disease (www.chestnet.org). Usually requires postgraduate training through the fellowship, several years' experience, and sub-specialty board certification.

(continued)

Table 27   Continued

FAAI	Your physician is a Fellow of the American Academy of Allergy, Asthma, and Immunology (www.aaaai.org), a professional society. Usually requires postgraduate training through the fellowship, several years' experience, and sub-specialty board certification.
PC	The designation P.C. after your physician's name is not a medical honor or qualification. It is a legal designation. The initials stand for Professional Corporation and indicate that the physician has formed a legal corporation and has filed articles of incorporation with the state.

osteopathy. Allopathic medicine has existed for centuries. Andrew Taylor Still founded the discipline of osteopathic medicine less than 150 years ago, in 1874. The philosophy of osteopathic medicine differs from the allopathic. Osteopathy seeks to treat the whole patient and emphasizes the importance of the musculoskeletal system, as well as the importance of osteopathic manipulative treatment. In the past, requirements for admission to an osteopathic medical school were considered to be less stringent than for admission to an allopathic medical school, but that has changed. The curricula of both schools are quite similar, and state licensing authorities, as well as most hospitals, recognize the M.D. and the D.O. degrees as equivalent.

After medical school, internship, residency, and fellowship training, qualified specialist physicians in the United States are permitted to take national, specialized examinations called board examinations. Successful candidates are then said to be board certified in their field, for example, in pulmonary medicine, or in allergy and immunology. Board certification indicates that the physician has met stringent training and testing qualifications.

Osteopathy

A system of medicine that uses conventional medical remedies and is based on the theory that disturbances in the musculoskeletal system affect other body parts and lead to disease. Consequently, manipulation of the body and musculoskeletal system restores health.

Many asthma specialists also enjoy teaching medical students, interns, residents, and fellows, and choose to become members of a medical school faculty.

General pediatricians, who take care of the majority of children with asthma, are experienced in asthma treatment, but are not technically true asthma specialists because they have not completed the specialized training described in this answer. The same is true for family practitioners and general adult internists who treat adults with asthma.

The best way to ascertain whether your treating physician specializes in asthma treatment is to ask the doctor directly. Make sure that your asthma physician is primarily a clinician or a doctor who takes care of patients for a living. Some lung physicians are more accurately described as physician-scientists. Although trained in respiratory medicine or allergy, they spend the great majority of their professional life in the laboratory, advancing our understanding and knowledge of the scientific aspects of asthma. Such physician-scientists might, for example, develop a new medication for asthma treatment or research the way asthma genes are transmitted. They are asthma specialists. They advance the knowledge of asthma, but are not involved with the direct delivery of healthcare. The concept of specialization thus includes not only sophisticated medical training beyond that of a general doctor, but also a real and abiding interest in asthma and in caring for people with asthma.

45. Do I need to consult a physician who specializes in asthma?

Referral to an asthma specialist is advised under two general circumstances: the "tricky" diagnosis, and the need for expert evaluation or treatment (Table 28).

Pediatrician

A physician specialized in the care of children and adolescents younger than 18 years of age. Pediatricians have received training in well-baby and well-child care as well as in the diagnosis and treatment of illnesses that can affect children from birth through adolescence.

Family practitioner

A type of physician specialized in the treatment of persons of all ages. May be qualified to perform minor surgical procedures, set fractures, and deliver babies in addition to providing medical care and prescribing medicines.

Internist

A physician specialized in the nonsurgical medical care of adults.

Table 28   When to Consult an Asthma Specialist

To establish the diagnosis

- If your "asthma" symptoms and signs are not typical of asthma, you should obtain a referral to an asthma specialist.
- If you require specialized diagnostic testing, you should obtain a referral to an expert. Examples of specialized diagnostic tests are allergy skin testing, rhinoscopy, complete pulmonary function studies, bronchoprovocation (Methacholine) challenge lung testing, and bronchoscopy.
- If it is suspected that an occupational or environmental inhalant is provoking or contributing to asthma (suspected occupational asthma or work-related asthma), you should obtain a referral to an asthma specialist.

To optimize treatment

- If you have experienced a serious, life-threatening asthma exacerbation, you should obtain a referral to an asthma specialist.
- If treatment of your asthma has required more than two bursts of oral corticosteroids in the past year or if you have experienced an exacerbation requiring hospitalization, you should obtain a referral to an asthma specialist.
- If you are not meeting the goals of asthma therapy after 3–6 months of treatment, you should obtain a referral to an asthma specialist.
- If your asthma remains poorly controlled with frequent exacerbations despite your adherence to appropriate asthma treatment, you should obtain a referral to an asthma specialist.
- If you have been diagnosed with other medical conditions that are known to potentially complicate the diagnosis and treatment of asthma, you should obtain a referral to an asthma specialist. Examples of such diagnoses include (but are not limited to) COPD, GERD, nasal polyps, severe allergic rhinitis, sinusitis, and VCD.
- If you require additional education about asthma and its treatment, guidance regarding possible complications of therapy, strategies on how to improve your adherence to treatments, including medications, monitoring, and allergen avoidance, you should obtain a referral to an asthma specialist.
- If you are being considered for immunotherapy ("allergy shots"), you should obtain a referral to an allergy and asthma specialist.
- If you require daily use of medium (or higher) dosing of ICS and a LABA (step 4 care or higher) to control your asthma, you should obtain a referral to an asthma specialist. Referral may be considered if you are on a low dose of ICS (step 3 care). Children younger than 4 years of age should be referred when treatment mandates a medium dosage of ICS (step 3 care) and referral may be considered for children on a low dosage of ICS (step 2 care).

Source: Modified and adapted from the 2007 NAEPP's *EPR-3*.

In the first circumstance, asthma might be a suspected yet unproven diagnosis, either because of atypical symptoms or because of a superimposed illness, and referral leads to resolution of a diagnostic puzzle. In the second circumstance, referral leads to improved asthma control.

Studies suggest that about 5% of adults with asthma are resistant to therapy as their asthma remains poorly controlled with frequent exacerbations despite appropriate treatment. It is not understood why this minority of adult patients do not fully respond to asthma therapy, although it has been observed as a group; they tend to have a higher rate of superimposed illnesses, such as GERD, severe allergic rhinitis, and psychiatric conditions. So-called difficult-to-control asthma can reflect a myriad of factors, from adverse socioeconomic circumstances to a rare form of corticosteroid-resistant asthma.

The decision to seek care from an asthma specialist can be a matter of patient preference but is more frequently a consequence of severity of disease.

In the United States, the majority of individuals with asthma receive their care from physicians who are generalist doctors, such as family practitioners, internists, and pediatricians. The decision to seek care from an asthma specialist can be a matter of patient preference but is more frequently a consequence of severity of disease. Consultation from an asthma specialist is indicated and appropriate when a person's asthma is not well controlled. An example is someone who has daily symptoms, frequent absences from work or school, or who requires hospitalization for asthma despite good adherence to a treatment plan. Similarly, persons with asthma classified as having moderate or severe persistent asthma should receive their care from an asthma specialist.

Consultation from an asthma specialist is indicated and appropriate when a person's asthma is not well controlled.

The most recent update of the NAEPP's *Expert Panel Report* (2007) addresses the question of when referral to an asthma specialist is mandatory and when it should be considered. Any person with asthma who has experienced a life-threatening exacerbation must be referred for consultation to an asthma specialist. The same is true if a person with asthma has required more than two bursts of oral corticosteroid treatments (pills) in the prior 12 months or has been hospitalized overnight with exacerbated asthma. Any adult with severe persistent asthma, or any patient who requires step 4 or higher asthma treatment, should be under the care of a physician with an expertise in clinical asthma management. Similarly, referral to an asthma specialist may be considered for adults with moderate persistent asthma requiring step 3 treatment. If immunotherapy treatment (allergy shots) is contemplated, then consultation with an allergist is mandatory.

46. How can I find out whether or not I have allergies? If I do have allergies in addition to my asthma, what types of treatment are available?

A strong link between asthma and allergy has been recognized for a long time and both diagnoses frequently co-exist, as explained in Question 9. Many people believe that they may be allergic to certain foods or aeroallergens, such as pollens or dog dander, for example. An astute observer might notice that after exposure to the suspected agent, an allergic symptom, such as itchy, watery eyes, nasal stuffiness, or throat tingling develops. At the other extreme, a person might be allergic and not make the connection, not recognizing the allergy symptoms for what they are. Sometimes, the treating physician may come to suspect that a recurrent group of symptoms outside of the lungs or that persistent asthma reflects an underlying allergy. In each circumstance, consultation with an allergy specialist or allergist can be extremely helpful and is highly recommended in order to determine whether an allergy is present or not.

Persons, especially children, whose asthma is persistent (as per the NAEPP's 2007 classification) should be evaluated for the possibility of allergen-induced asthma. The most important allergens from an asthma perspective are inhaled allergens, including indoor allergens (such as dust mites, animal dander, and cockroaches) and outdoor fungal spores. Seasonal asthma has been linked with exposure to grass, ragweed, and pollen in sensitized persons. Food allergy does not typically precipitate asthma symptoms.

If your treating physician believes that you have significant symptoms of allergy, referral to an allergy specialist may be considered. Allergists are experts in evaluating and caring for children and adults who have allergic diseases. Evaluation always begins with a detailed history of the patient's symptoms and a review of the family history. The physical examination places particular emphasis on the skin, upper respiratory tract, and lungs. Important clues to diagnosing allergy often are found on close inspection of the skin, eyes, throat, and nasal passages, and on auscultation of the lungs. An attentive physician can therefore detect various specific findings of allergy if they are present on the physical examination. After obtaining a complete history and performing a physical examination, the next step in the evaluation may require specific allergy testing. Testing is performed either directly on the skin (in vivo allergy testing) or as a laboratory procedure (in vitro allergy testing) with a blood sample.

Direct testing refers to one of two techniques, sometimes collectively called skin testing. The first uses the prick puncture method and is performed on the skin of the patient's forearm or back. The prick puncture form of testing thus does not involve receiving an injection. If the result of the prick puncture test is not definitive, then the next step in the evaluation of suspected allergy may require intradermal tests, typically on the upper arm. An intradermal test requires a very superficial injection directly into the skin layer. Indirect testing

Allergist

A physician specialized in the diagnosis and treatment of persons with allergies.

Allergy testing

Methods of diagnosing allergies. Allergy tests can be obtained by two general methods: either directly on the patient or indirectly through a blood sample (RAST or ImmunoCAP) drawn from a vein.

(in vitro) requires venipuncture, during which a sample (tube) of blood from a vein is obtained through a needle stick. The first commercially introduced in vitro allergy test, developed by Pharmacia Diagnostics of Uppsala Sweden, was named RAST (which stands for RadioAllergoSorbent Test) and became widely available by the mid-1970s. The company developed a more refined test in 1989 called ImmunoCAP, which has now supplanted the first-generation RAST.

A "positive allergy" test result reflects prior exposure followed by sensitization to the specific allergen tested. The positive test result indicates that the immune system has been stimulated to produce a protein, namely an IgE antibody specifically directed against the tested allergen. Consider for example a college student who each year when he moves into his dorm at school in the late summer, notices several weeks of nasal congestion, cough, and a flare of his typical asthma symptoms requiring a step up in asthma medication. His allergist suspects a ragweed allergy. Direct testing with ragweed extract is positive, which means that our college student's immune system has over time been stimulated to produce an IgE antibody (see the next question for more information on IgE) directed against ragweed. Our student sensitized to ragweed is now "primed" to have an allergic reaction when again exposed to ragweed. When he returns to college during ragweed season, he experiences nasal symptoms and his asthma flares as a consequence of his ragweed allergy.

Many mistakenly believe that blood testing (RAST or ImmunoCAP) is somehow more accurate than direct allergy testing in evaluation of allergy. RAST is a valid technique for determining allergic sensitivity and the presence of IgE antibodies. The ImmunoCAP provides additional detailed measurement of IgE antibody levels.

In vitro

A process carried out outside of a living organism, in a man-made environment such as a test tube or culture medium. Any test or experiment performed in a laboratory would be considered an in vitro test. Derived from the Latin word for in glass.

RadioAllergo-Sorbent Test (RAST)

A trademark of Pharmacia Diagnostics that originated and developed the first RAST. It is a laboratory allergy test that detects and measures the level of IgE antibodies directed against specific antigens in a blood sample. Measuring blood RAST is one way of assessing the possible presence of an allergy.

Sensitization

In the context of allergy, the process by which a person becomes, over time, increasingly allergic to a substance (sensitizer) through repeated exposure to that substance.

Antibody

A protein molecule produced in blood or in tissues in direct response to a foreign substance or antigen. A specific antigen leads to the production of a corresponding specific antibody. The production of antibody can be beneficial or deleterious, depending on the circumstances.

In vivo

Allergy tests performed by prick/puncture or intradermal technique on a patient. A term derived from the Latin meaning within a living being.

Antihistamine

The class of medicines that counteract the effects of histamine by blocking histamine receptors on cells, which, in turn, prevents symptoms such as sneezing, runny nose, or watering eyes. Antihistamines are most effective when taken before symptoms develop.

Specific clinical situations may lead an allergist to recommend an in vitro (blood) method of testing rather than in vivo, recognizing, too, that in vivo (skin testing) requires specific skill and experience to perform. Persons with active skin conditions, such as eczema or psoriasis, or very reactive skin are not appropriate candidates for direct allergy (skin) testing and are better evaluated with a blood test, for instance. A very young child and anyone who has an exaggerated fear of needles would be possible candidates for RAST testing as well. Finally, a person who requires daily antihistamine medication that cannot be temporarily discontinued should be considered for blood testing, since allowing direct (in vivo) skin testing yields unreliable results if a person is taking antihistamine medication at the time of testing. Testing for many different suspected food allergies in a young child can be performed effectively all at once with the RAST or ImmunoCAP blood test.

Once the diagnosis of a specific allergy (or allergies) is established, the next step is initiating appropriate treatment. There are three basic and complementary approaches to the treatment of allergic diseases: allergen avoidance, medication, and immunotherapy. The first measure is to avoid contact with and exposure to the allergen whenever possible. Some allergens, such as foods, can generally be passed up by careful menu planning and close review of food labels, while others, like tree pollen, cannot reasonably be entirely avoided, and some (like an adored family pet) might be extremely difficult to stay away from. Even so, it is also important for a person with allergy to have as normal and healthy a lifestyle as possible. If you are allergic to an environmental allergen (such as a cat, dog, or hamster) and you consistently and reliably implement successful environmental allergen control, you may not require any medication or further treatment.

Environmental control alone is not however always sufficient in treating significant allergy. Despite excellent
environmental control and determined efforts at allergen
avoidance, additional measures are usually required for
optimal allergy treatment. The second strategy in allergy
treatment is the prescription of appropriate medications
(pharmacotherapy) to effectively control symptoms. Note,
however, that the medications prescribed for control of
allergy symptoms cannot cure the underlying allergy.
Immunotherapy, commonly referred to as "allergy shots,"
is the third approach employed for the treatment of allergic asthma and is the only method of treatment that has
the potential to "turn down," or possibly turn off, the ability of the immune system to react to specific allergens. If
there is no allergic reaction, there will be no asthma symptoms. Consider, for instance, a patient with documented
tree and grass pollen allergies whose parents came to an
allergist seeking a second opinion when he was 11 years
old. He had first developed allergy symptoms in first
grade. Over the next 4 years, and despite excellent compliance with antihistamine pills, nasal allergy sprays, and
environmental controls such as use of air conditioning
and air filters, this youngster experienced worsening allergic symptoms every spring and summer. Immediately
before he was brought in for his consultation, he required
several courses of oral corticosteroid medication over the
course of a single spring and summer season. One of our
treatment recommendations included consideration of
immunotherapy directed against tree and grass allergens.
This patient proceeded with immunotherapy and is now
an active, sports-loving 16-year-old who no longer
needs to use nasal steroid sprays and daily antihistamines in order to function. During the allergy season—
spring into early summer—he takes only an infrequent
antihistamine to control his markedly reduced symptoms. Participation in his favorite sports—soccer and

*Environmen-
tal control
alone is not
however
always suffi-
cient in treat-
ing significant
allergy.*

**Environmental
control**

The avoidance or
elimination from the
home, school, or work
environment of those
substances, allergens,
or irritants that are
responsible for a
patient's symptoms.

Pharmacotherapy

Treatment by med-
ication administered
either by mouth,
through injection,
inhalation, or
intravenously.

Immunotherapy

One of the three
main therapeutic
approaches to the
management of
allergic disorders.
Various terms have
been used to describe
this form of therapy,
including desensiti-
zation (which is a
misnomer), hyposen-
sitization, or, most
commonly, allergy
shots.

Asthma: Treatment Plans, Goals, and Strategies

baseball—no longer presents the challenges it did before he started his allergy treatments. Immunotherapy directed against tree and grass pollens has caused his immune system to turn down and almost turn off his ability to react allergically to either of these pollen classes. With continued therapy, it would not be unreasonable for this young man to be rid of his allergic sensitivity to the spring-season pollens.

Immunotherapy has been proven effective in the treatment of selected persons with allergic asthma, allergic rhinitis, and insect sting allergy.

Allergists are physicians who are experts in administering immunotherapy. Immunotherapy has been proven effective in the treatment of selected persons with allergic asthma, allergic rhinitis, and insect sting allergy. Treatment initially requires weekly visits and lasts for an average of 3–5 years but sometimes more. Over time, the interval between injection visits extends to 3–4 weeks during the maintenance phase. The 2007 NAEPP's *EPR-3* advises that immunotherapy be considered for any person with persistent asthma "if evidence is clear of a relationship between symptoms and exposure to an allergen to which the patient is sensitive."

Kerrin's comment:

We had my son tested for allergies when he was 2 years old. We were especially concerned about a peanut allergy because he had a reaction to a cookie someone brought from a bakery that we suspected had either been made with peanut oil or had come in contact with peanut ingredients. The allergy specialist performed a test on his back because he was too young to be certain he would not wipe off the serum. The hardest part was keeping him still for the 20 minutes it took for the test to complete. But they had a VCR in the office and he quickly settled down. And the test showed that he had a severe peanut allergy, so the very short discomfort was a small price to pay for knowing this potentially life-saving piece of information.

47. What is immunoglobulin E (IgE)?

Immunoglobulins are protein molecules that circulate in the bloodstream. They are part of the body's immune response to a stimulus perceived as foreign, such as bacteria, parasites, or allergens. There are five classes of immunoglobulins, named G, A, M, E, and D, and abbreviated: IgG, IgA, IgM, IgE, and IgD. Each class has its own characteristics. IgE is an immunoglobulin whose levels in the body rise in certain situations, including in the setting of an allergic response. Persons with allergy and asthma will often demonstrate elevated IgE blood levels as compared to a normal individual with neither allergy nor asthma. IgE plays an important, central role in several allergic conditions, namely asthma, allergic rhinitis, atopic dermatitis (also known as eczema), certain food allergies (e.g., peanuts and fish), urticaria (hives), and anaphylaxis. Recent understanding of the pivotal role of IgE has led directly to the development of a novel medication that blocks the effects of IgE, as discussed in Question 72. By blocking IgE, the allergic response is lessened or eliminated, offering promising treatment of asthma and severe food allergies.

48. My asthma is active; how do I know whether I should go to the nearest hospital emergency room?

Gemma's comment:

Emergencies can be scary. During a vacation at a popular seaside resort in the northeast, I was caught on the beach as a squall came up, blowing sand in my face and mouth.

Immunoglobulin

A protein produced by the body's immune system as part of an immune response to an antigen. Antigens can be infectious agents such as viruses, bacteria and parasites, or other proteins.

Immunoglobulin E (IgE)

A type of immunoglobulin that rises and is produced by the body in greater quantity in the setting of atopy, allergic asthma, and a typical allergic reaction.

Urticaria

The scientific name for hives, a type of skin rash. Urticaria are raised, welt-like, reddened, and intensely itchy. The most common cause of urticaria is an allergic reaction.

Anaphylaxis

The most severe form of an allergic reaction or response. If untreated, anaphylaxis can be fatal. The term *anaphylactic shock* is sometimes used to describe the most dramatic and serious form of anaphylaxis. Anaphylaxis usually involves several organ systems, including the cardiovascular system, the skin, the respiratory system, and the gastrointestinal tract.

Because my children were playing happily, I delayed leaving the beach, and by the time I did, I was gasping for breath, almost unable to climb up the dunes. By the time I got to an emergency room later that evening, my breathing was very labored. The treatment was scary, too. I was given a shot of adrenaline, which made breathing easy, and sent home. The adrenaline kept me wired (i.e., extremely tense and unable to sleep) for more than a day. I should add that this emergency occurred 20 years ago, and that I was treated in a small regional hospital, better prepared to deal with boating accidents than breathing problems. I'm sure the treatment would be better today.

The inability to gain control of an asthma exacerbation is the major reason for proceeding to the nearest hospital for emergency treatment (Table 29). The simple fact that your asthma is more active might not in itself warrant an emergency room visit. If your asthma responds to increased treatment as advocated in the NAEPP's guidelines, or as outlined in your asthma care plan, then you might simply need to check in with your asthma provider. If your asthma symptoms do not respond to the increased treatment, or if your symptoms worsen despite such treatment, then a visit to the emergency room is indicated. The decision to proceed to the emergency room is based on medical considerations as well as common sense. Keep in mind that each individual's asthma is unique. Some individuals may experience rapidly worsening exacerbations, for example, and the rate of how rapidly your asthma tends to progress should certainly be taken into account as well.

I always remind my patients that emergency rooms are open and staffed 24 hours a day for a reason—because they are needed!

I always remind my patients that emergency rooms are open and staffed 24 hours a day for a reason—because they are needed! Asthma unresponsive to stepped-up home treatment is exactly the type of condition that

Table 29   Serious Signs and Symptoms of Exacerbated Asthma

Make sure you and your asthma healthcare provider have a plan for asthma emergencies. Keep important phone numbers handy.

The worrisome asthma symptoms that follow warrant seeking emergency medical care immediately. Asthma healthcare providers may instruct their patients to begin steroid treatment at the first suspicion of an asthma emergency.

Children and Adults	Babies and Young Children
Marked breathlessness	**Noisy, raspy breathing**
• Difficulty speaking in full sentences	**Cough**
• Difficulty walking	**Fast breathing**
• Tight chest	**Fussy behavior**
• Feels winded	**Sits upright, won't lie down**
Labored breathing	**Difficult to feed; can't eat or drink because of breathing**
• Shoulders rise with breathing	
• Neck and ribs move inward with breathing	**Nostrils flare with breathing**
• Rapid, uncomfortable breaths	**Neck moves inward when breathing**
• Cough, day and/or night	**Ribs move inward while breathing**
• Wheezing	**Discolored blue-gray skin near mouth**
Altered mentation	**Medicines aren't effective**
• Difficulty thinking clearly	
• Confusion, loss of alertness	
Lowered oxygen	
• Gray or blue lips	
• Gray or blue fingertips	
Low PEF values	
• PEF < 60% personal best	
Medicines "Not Working"	
• PEF fails to rise after using "quick-relief" medicine	
• Symptoms continue	

emergency rooms are designed to treat. The key is not to hesitate to proceed to the emergency room if your asthma specialist advises you to, or if the protocol you're following as part of your asthma action plan calls for it. Every asthma action plan must include clear criteria for when you must obtain emergency care. A red-zone peak expiratory flow (PEF) less than 50% of your personal best is a clear-cut indicator of worsening asthma and warrants transportation to the emergency room. Don't delay! Trying to tough it out will only make it harder to control your exacerbation. It is better to intervene early and quickly. Consider, as part of your routine asthma care, discussing ahead of time with your asthma doctor how best to handle increased asthma symptoms, when to start steroid therapy, when to telephone for advice, and when to go to the emergency room.

Kerrin's comment:

When my son had his first respiratory episode, we didn't know what was happening. He had a cold, he had a very productive-sounding cough, and he was wheezing. We had the nebulizer from an earlier illness he had during which his doctor heard wheezes, although nothing as extreme as what we were hearing this time. We used the nebulizer, which worked for a short time, but only a couple of hours. We had to re-treat him within 2 hours. We put him to bed after one of the treatments and he seemed to be doing better, but after checking on him an hour later we thought he might be having trouble again. It was hard to tell, though, because he was asleep; we couldn't really see the retractions in his chest, and we thought perhaps his deep breathing was just from the fact that he was asleep. When we called the doctor, she asked us to hold the phone up to his mouth so she could hear him, and she told us to look at his neck to see if retractions were occurring there; they were, and they were very obvious. Hearing this, combined with the fact that we were having to readminister treatments within 4 hours, she told us to take him straight to the hospital. He ended up having to stay for 2 days.

Retraction

A sucking in or visible depression of the muscles in the spaces between the ribs that occurs with labored breathing.

49. What kind of emergency treatment can I expect when I get to the emergency room?

The actual treatment you receive in the emergency department of the hospital depends on the individual characteristics of your asthma, other health conditions you may have, as well as the severity of your symptoms when you arrive in the emergency room. In general, you can expect three components to your emergency care. The first will consist of immediate treatment with supplemental oxygen, bronchodilators, and anti-inflammatory medicines to gain control of the asthma exacerbation. The second component to your care will consist of careful assessment of the degree of asthma severity, along with close monitoring of your condition and overall response to treatment. The third component will determine whether any other superimposed conditions are present and how they might affect your asthma.

You can expect to be given supplemental oxygen to breathe, via either nasal prongs or a mask, as mentioned in Question 43. You will likely be given repeated doses of short-acting β_2 inhaled bronchodilator therapy in succession by a nebulizer or MDI (metered-dose inhaler) with a valved holding chamber (VHC). A temporary intravenous catheter (IV) may be inserted into a vein in your arm to allow for rapid administration of fluids to counter any dehydration. Steroids in pill form or via the IV (if already placed) will be prescribed to reduce airway inflammation. Other inhaled treatments and intravenous medicine may be prescribed on a case-by-case basis. As your treatment gets under way, you will be examined with close attention to vital signs and the lung exam. Your pulse and oxygen level will likely be monitored by a special sensor called a pulse oximeter, described in Question 43. The pulse oximeter clips onto your fingertip and is painless. You may be asked to wear a heart monitor, which is made up of thin wires attached to electrodes stuck to the skin of the chest on one end and connected to a monitor screen on the other. The emergency room doctor and nurse assigned to your care will keep watch on you as you receive the prescribed treatments. Some hospitals also have respiratory therapists on duty in the emergency room, and they will certainly play a role in your care as well. You will be asked to perform serial peak-flow measurements to help gauge your response to treatment.

You can expect to spend at least 4 hours undergoing emergency treatment of asthma. You may undergo a chest X-ray and blood tests if an infection is suspected. You may be asked if you know what triggered your asthma. Under the ideal circumstances, your exacerbation will become controlled in the emergency room, and your asthma will be stabilized. Your symptoms will lessen, and your peak flow will rise into a safe zone and remain there during your emergency room stay. You will be given specific instructions for stepped-up asthma care, and you will need to contact and see your regular asthma doctor for a visit within a few days of the emergency room visit. If, on the other hand, your exacerbation cannot be controlled within 6–12 hours of aggressive management, you will likely be admitted to the hospital for continued care. If the physicians treating you in the emergency setting advise hospitalization, then agree. You must take their best medical advice, no matter how inconvenient it may seem! The worst case scenario consists of an individual who misjudges the severity of an exacerbation and waits too long for treatment, or who doesn't follow recommendations and ends up with out-of-control asthma that can lead to respiratory failure, and tragically, albeit rarely, even death.

50. Is it true that a person can die of asthma?

Yes, asthma can be fatal. Thousands of people die each year in the United States from uncontrolled asthma. Asthma is a highly treatable disease. Death from asthma is especially tragic because each one of those deaths is theoretically 100% preventable. Analysis of recent trends in the United States suggests that after decades of increasing, the number of deaths from asthma appears to have leveled off and is beginning to decrease.

In 2001, there were 4269 reported deaths from asthma in the United States—more than 11 deaths a day! The 4055 recorded deaths from asthma in 2003 suggested a downward trend, which was further supported by data that are more recent. By 2006, the reported death rate from asthma was 1.2 per 100,000 population, corresponding to the fact that 3613 persons died of asthma in the United States that year. The statistics further reveal that asthma deaths are rare in children and that the highest death rate from asthma was in Puerto Ricans. According to the CDC, "Puerto Ricans were the most likely to die from asthma and had asthma death rates 360% higher than non-Hispanic white people. Non-Hispanic black people had an asthma death rate 200% higher than non-Hispanic white people did. Females had an asthma death rate 45% higher than males." Despite the encouraging trends, the statistics remain shocking; it indicates that on average, almost ten individuals die from asthma each day in the United States. These deaths occur at a time when science has made enormous strides in the understanding of asthma. Never before has healthcare been so sophisticated. Never before has the medical profession had access to such highly effective, safe medications and treatments for asthma. Yet, undiagnosed and inadequately treated asthma continues to represent a significant public health burden. Every single asthma death is a failure at one or multiple levels. One such common failure is ignoring new or increasing asthma symptoms, for example. Experts have turned their attention to factors responsible for fatal asthma, as detailed in the next question.

51. What are the characteristics of fatal or near-fatal asthma?

Fatal and near-fatal asthma have been the subject of much interest and study. By obtaining as much information as possible on persons who die or almost die of asthma, we can learn how to prevent similar deaths in the future (see Table 30).

The majority of persons with near-fatal or fatal asthma tend to underestimate the severity of their symptoms and

Table 30   Fatal Asthma: Risk Factors

- Prior history of sudden, rapidly progressive severe exacerbations
- Prior history of intubation for asthma, ever
- Prior history of admission to an intensive care unit (ICU) for asthma, ever
- Two or more hospitalizations for asthma in the last 12 months
- Three or more visits to a hospital emergency room for asthma exacerbation in the last 12 months
- Either an emergency room visit or a hospitalization for asthma in the last 30 days
- Asthma requiring the use of two (or more) canisters of rescue quick-relief short-acting β_2 agonist inhalers in the last 30 days
- Current requirement for and use of oral (pill form) steroid medication
- Recent steroid taper
- Allergy or sensitivity to mold (Alternaria test)
- Lack of awareness of worsening asthma; difficulty in perceiving worsening asthma symptoms
- Other superimposed complicating serious medical illnesses (heart disease, diabetes, etc.)
- Serious psychiatric illness
- Severe psychosocial problems
- Lower socioeconomic status
- Urban residence
- Illicit "recreational" drug use and/or abuse

present for care only after several days of clearly worsening symptoms. The symptoms are usually responses to triggers that can include a viral infection, intense exposure to allergens, nonadherence to prescribed asthma treatment, air pollution, changes in weather, or severe emotional stress. If someone waits for a period of days before intervening to control the exacerbation, the opportunity for effective treatment is lost; in other words, it is too late by the time help is on the way. In most cases of fatal or near-fatal asthma, the actual disease can be controlled, but human patient factors adversely modify the outcome.

The more unusual scenario of very rapidly progressive asthma that exacerbates dramatically over the course of several hours occurs in the minority of patients with near-fatal or fatal asthma. Some individuals have a particularly aggressive and severe type of asthma that, despite ideal and perfect compliance with medical treatment and recommendations, does lead to severe complications. Those persons should be under the care of an asthma specialist and may be candidates for cutting-edge therapies.

In most cases of fatal or near-fatal asthma, the actual disease can be controlled, but human patient factors adversely modify the outcome.

52. What is respiratory failure?

Respiratory failure develops when the lungs and respiratory system become unable to provide the body with sufficient oxygen (O_2) and fail to excrete or "blow off" accumulated carbon dioxide (CO_2). When the major disturbance is primarily an inability of the respiratory system to meet the body's oxygen (O_2) requirements, then hypoxemic respiratory failure is present. When CO_2 and acid levels rise within the body because the lungs are unable to keep up their excretory function, then hypercarbic respiratory failure occurs. A mixed hypoxemic and hypercarbic pattern may exist.

Respiratory failure can be very gradual, and it may develop and progress slowly over time, from months to years, as in the case of chronic respiratory failure. Progressive cigarette-related emphysema is one example of a cause of gradual respiratory insufficiency that may, with time, continue on to respiratory failure. Asthma is not typically a cause of chronic respiratory failure. Acute respiratory failure, as the name implies, occurs rapidly over a period of hours to days.

Fatal or near-fatal asthma, thankfully rare events, are both causes of acute respiratory failure. In either situation, acute or chronic, there comes a point where the respiratory failure becomes so marked that the body will become deprived of adequate oxygen and be subjected to dangerously rising levels of carbon dioxide and acids. Sampling of arterial blood gases (ABGs) in fatal and near-fatal asthma, for example, show low values of oxygen (the PaO_2 value is <60 mmHg) and rising levels of carbon dioxide (the $PaCO_2$ value rises above 41 mmHg). As the lungs no longer function effectively and fail, other organs will begin to fail in response. The brain, in particular, is very sensitive to low oxygen levels, as well as to elevations in carbon dioxide values, each of which are harmful separately. As the oxygen and carbon dioxide levels become more abnormal, consciousness becomes impaired. Coma and death will ensue. An individual with progressive respiratory failure is usually critically ill and in danger of death without aggressive medical intervention and life support, as reviewed in more detail in Question 53.

Endotracheal intubation

The procedure in which a specialized breathing tube is placed into the trachea through the mouth or the nasal passages to allow airway support and the administration of extra oxygen.

53. What is endotracheal intubation?

Endotracheal intubation is performed in the setting of respiratory failure due to any cause, including respiratory failure from asthma. It is a potentially life-saving medical intervention. Patients who require endotracheal intubation are critically ill, because their lungs are unable to take in oxygen and exhale carbon dioxide. The intubation procedure itself can be performed in an emergency room, an intensive care unit, or out of hospital, in the field, provided the appropriate equipment and qualified medical personnel are available. Ambulance crews with advanced cardiac live support (ACLS) certification are trained in endotracheal intubation. The procedure itself consists of the temporary placement of a soft, flexible, plastic breathing tube through the nose or mouth, past the voice box (larynx), and into the trachea or main breathing tube.

Endotracheal intubation serves three major functions. First, it keeps a person's airway open in situations when it would otherwise close off, causing asphyxiation, such as in the case of decreasing levels of consciousness. Second, it also allows for the removal, by suctioning, of any mucus that has accumulated in the airways. Third, and perhaps most importantly, endotracheal intubation allows a doctor to provide the intubated patient with breaths and extra oxygen to inhale, thus taking over the work of breathing from failing lungs. In order to take over a person's breathing, the end of the endotracheal tube is connected to a ventilator. A ventilator is a machine that is designed to provide individualized support to a patient in respiratory failure. The support provided by the ventilator consists of breaths along with supplemental oxygen. Once ventilator support is initiated, then the focus shifts to treatment of the underlying cause of the respiratory failure. The goal is to reverse the process that led to a need for intubation. If lung function thus returns and there is no longer a need to assist breathing, then the endotracheal tube is easily removed.

Larynx

The voice box. Two vocal cords allow for speech as inhaled air passes between them and sets up vibrations within the larynx located in the middle of the neck.

PART FIVE

Asthma: Inhaled Medications and Advances

What medications are useful in treating asthma?

Will I need to take asthma medicine forever?

Why are so many asthma medicines in inhaler form?

What is the correct way to use my dry-powder inhaler (DPI)?

What is the correct way to use my metered-dose inhaler (MDI)?

What are corticosteroids and how do they work in asthma?

More . . .

54. What medications are useful in treating asthma?

Different classes of medicines are useful in the treatment of asthma. The NAEPP's asthma classification helps define the severity of a person's asthma and assists in guiding therapy. Notice that for each asthma classification, the NAEPP makes specific suggestions about the best type of medicine to use for treating that specific level of asthma.

Asthma medicines are best prescribed in a stepwise approach. The physician initiates treatment with one or two types of medicine, based on the patient's initial degree of asthma severity and then adds or reduces medication based on the patient's symptom control, lung function, and overall state of well-being. A person with intermittent asthma might be instructed to use a short-acting β_2 inhaler as needed for symptom relief. With the onset of winter and colder temperatures, that individual's symptoms may start to become more prominent and increase. The inhaled, short-acting β_2 medicine that formerly kept asthma symptoms under control might be required several times daily. No longer intermittent, this patient's asthma has "moved up" a classification to become mild persistent asthma. Just as the classification has moved up, the treatment is stepped up or intensified. For this patient, an additional, second medication with anti-inflammatory properties, such as an inhaled steroid in low doses, would be a good choice (Table 31). Once good asthma control is achieved with the combination of an inhaled anti-inflammatory and a β_2 bronchodilator, and after the improvement is sustained for at least three months, it would then be appropriate to consider a step down, especially if the stimulus to stepped-up asthma has resolved (such as the end of cold winter weather).

Table 31 Asthma Medication Facts

Short-Acting β_2 Agonist (SABA) bronchodilators: albuterol (called salbutamol outside the United States), levalbuterol, pirbuterol are as needed, quick-relief asthma medicines.

- All persons with asthma need a prescription for an inhaled SABA.
- Inhaled SABAs are prescribed for fast symptom relief, and used only when and as needed.
- Inhaled SABAs are the most effective therapy for rapid reversal of symptoms of bronchoconstriction.
- Inhaled SABAs have an onset of action of 5 minutes or less.
- Inhaled SABAs have a peak effect 30 to 60 minutes after inhalation.
- Inhaled SABAs' effects on bronchoconstriction last for 4 to 6 hours.
- When inhaling two puffs of a SABA, you should wait 10–15 seconds between puffs.

Inhaled Corticosteroids (ICS)

- Any person with asthma that is persistent (mild, moderate, or severe persistent) should use an ICS every day. The dose will vary depending on the extent of asthma.
- ICSs are the cornerstone of preventive therapy in all forms of persistent asthma.
- ICSs reduce and suppress inflammation in the airways and so prevent asthma symptoms.
- ICSs are daily-use controller medicines.
- Daily ICS use results in improved asthma outcomes and improved quality of life.
- Many physicians (and therefore their patients) do not follow national guidelines such as the NAEPP for ICS prescribing in asthma.
- Long-acting β_2 agonist bronchodilators should never be used without simultaneous anti-inflammatory medication, such as ICS.

Asthma treatment must take into account the often fluid and changeable character of asthma itself.

A useful and practical way of classifying asthma medicines is by their method of action. In such a schema, the two major categories of medicine used in asthma treatment are quick-relief, fast-acting medicines and long-term control medicines (Table 32). Quick-relief asthma medicines have a prompt onset of action and act rapidly to relieve airway narrowing (bronchoconstriction). You may know them as "reliever" or "rescue" medications. They include the short-acting β_2 agonist bronchodilators, or SABA, inhaled anticholinergics, and oral (pill or liquid)

Asthma treatment must take into account the often fluid and changeable character of asthma itself.

Table 32 Medications Used in Asthma Treatment: A Classification

Daily Use Long-term Control Medications	Quick-relief, Rapid-acting Medications
Inhaled corticosteroids • Beclomethasone • Budesonide • Flunisolide • Fluticasone • Mometasone • Triamcinolone	Inhaled short-acting β_2 agonists • Albuterol • Levalbuterol • Pirbuterol
Inhaled cromolyn and nedocromil • Cromolyn • Nedocromil	Inhaled anticholinergics • Ipratropium (not currently FDA approved for asthma) • Tiotropium (not currently FDA approved for asthma)
Oral leukotriene modifiers • Montelukast • Zafirlukast • Zileuton	Oral corticosteroids for "bursts" • Methylprednisolone • Prednisone
Long-acting β_2 agonists (LABA) • Salmeterol • Formoterol	
Methylxanthines • Sustained release theophylline	
Immunomodulators • Omalizumab	

corticosteroid bursts. The long-term control asthma medicines must be taken daily to achieve control of asthma, and then to maintain that level of control. They are referred to interchangeably as "long-term preventive," "controller," or "maintenance" medications. They include the inhaled corticosteroids (Table 33), inhaled forms of cromolyn and nedocromil, leukotriene modifiers (Table 38), long-acting β_2 agonist bronchodilators, or LABA (Tables 35 and 36), theophylline, and anti-IgE immunomodulator medication.

Table 33   Inhaled Corticosteroid (ICS) Medications: Generic & Trade Names

Generic Name	Trade Name
Beclomethasone HFA	Qvar
Budesonide DPI	Pulmicort Flexhaler
Budesonide inhalation suspension	Pulmicort Respules
Ciclesonide	Alvesco HFA
Flunisolide	Aerobid, Aerobid-M
Flunisolide HFA	Aerospan HFA
Fluticasone HFA MDI	Flovent HFA
Fluticasone DPI	Flovent Diskus
Monometasone DPI	Asmanex
Triamcinolone	Azmacort

Table 34   Short-Acting β-Agonist (SABA) Bronchodilator Medications: Generic & Trade Names

Generic Name	Trade Name
• Albuterol HFA MDI • Albuterol solution for nebulization	• Ventolin HFA • ProAir • Proventil HFA • ReliOn Ventolin HFA • AccuNeb
• Levalbuterol HFA MDI • Levalbuterol solution for nebulization	• Xopenex HFA • Xopenex inhalation solution
• Pirbuterol	• Maxair

Persons with persistent asthma (mild, moderate, or severe persistent asthma) require treatment with medicine from each of the two broad classes of asthma medication, using both quick-relief medication and long-term control medicines for optimal asthma control. The actual medication and dosages are, of course, best selected by the treating physician. Individuals whose asthma is intermittent, according to the NAEPP classification and criteria, will

131

Table 35   Long-Acting β-Agonist (LABA) Bronchodilator Medications: Generic & Trade Names

Generic Name	Trade Name
Formoterol DPI	Foradil DPI
Salmeterol DPI	Serevent Diskus, Serevent DPI
Arformoterol solution for nebulization	Brovana*
Formoterol solution for nebulization	Performist*

*Note: The LABA solutions for inhalation through nebulization, Brovana and Performist, are as of this writing, FDA approved for the treatment of COPD, not for asthma.

Table 36   Combination of ICS & LABA Medications: Generic & Trade Names

Generic Name	Trade Name
Budesonide + formoterol	Symbicort HFA
Fluticasone + salmeterol	Advair HFA Advair Diskus

typically be prescribed a quick-relief medicine alone, such as a short-acting β_2 agonist bronchodilator (SABA) inhaled as needed for symptom relief.

Most asthma medicines are inhaled (Table 37). The inhaled route is preferred because it delivers the medicine directly into the breathing passages. Why take a pill form of a medicine that leads to measurable drug levels in the entire body when you can deposit effective medicine exactly where it's needed for quick symptom relief? In addition, side effects, if any, are minimal. Short-acting β_2 agents (SABA) like albuterol, levalbuterol, and pirbuterol in inhaled form are all examples of ideal, quick-relief medicines that relax smooth muscle and bronchodilate the breathing passages (Table 34). They are the therapy of choice for the relief of acute symptoms and for pre-exercise treatment in persons with EIB. Quick-relief or "rescue"

Albuterol

The generic name for a β_2 agonist medication that acts on the respiratory passages to cause bronchodilatation. It is classified as a quick-relief, fast-acting medicine and is extensively prescribed in the treatment of bronchial asthma.

Table 37   Asthma Medicines Delivered via Inhalers

Short-Acting, Quick-Relief β₂-Agonist Bronchodilators (SABA)

ProAir HFA (albuterol sulfate)

Proventil HFA (albuterol sulfate)

ReliOn Ventolin HFA (albuterol sulfate)

Ventolin HFA (albuterol sulfate)

Xopenex HFA (levalbuterol HCl)

Maxair Autohaler (pirbuterol acetate)

Daily Use Anti-Inflammatory Corticosteroids

Aerobid (flunisolide)

Aerospan HFA (flunisolide hemihydrate)

Alvesco HFA (ciclesonide)

Asmanex (mometasone furoate)

Azmacort (triamcinolone acetonide)

Flovent HFA (fluticasone propionate)

Pulmicort Flexhaler (budesonide)

Qvar (beclomethasone dipropionate)

Anti-Inflammatory and Anti-Allergy

Intal MDI (cromolyn sodium)—*no longer manufactured as MDI after 2009*

Tilade MDI (nedocromil sodium)—*no longer manufactured as MDI after 2008*

Combination Products

Advair (fluticasone propionate & salmeterol xinafoate)

Symbicort (budesonide & formoterol fumarate)

Long-Acting Daily Use β₂-Agonist Bronchodilators (LABA)

Foradil (formoterol fumarate)

Serevent (salmeterol xinafoate)

LABA should not be taken alone, but simultaneously with inhaled corticosteroids

---

inhalers are thus usually prescribed for use when needed. The onset of action is rapid, and the beneficial effects last between 4 and 6 hours. You should keep your quick-relief inhaler handy during the day. Keep it in a briefcase, pocket, purse, or gym bag. Like your house key, your quick-relief inhaler should accompany you wherever you go.

Like your house key, your quick-relief inhaler should accompany you wherever you go.

Table 38   Oral (pill-form) Leukotriene Modifier Medications: Generic & Trade Names

Generic Name	Trade Name
Montelukast *A leukotriene receptor antagonist—LTRA*	Singulair (*granules, chewable, tablets*)
Zafirlukast *A leukotriene receptor antagonist—LTRA*	Accolate
Zileuton *A leukotriene synthesis inhibitor*	Zyflo

Daily long-term asthma control medicines are used in addition to quick-relief medicine for treatment of the persistent forms of asthma: mild persistent, moderate persistent, and severe persistent. Controller medicines include both inhaled and oral preparations. The NAEPP recommends inhaled corticosteroids as first-line inhaled anti-inflammatory treatment and advocates their use beginning with mild persistent asthma (see Table 33). The leukotriene-modifier class of controller-asthma medicine is a newer type of controller medication (see Table 38). The group includes montelukast and zafirlukast, which are of the LTRA (leukotriene receptor antagonist) sub-class as well as a third drug, zileuton, which acts by a different mechanism (as a lipoxygenase pathway inhibitor). The two LTRAs are FDA approved for young children (montelukast for children over the age of 1 year, and zafirlukast for youngsters aged 7 years and older) in addition to adolescents and adults. Since montelukast requires once-a-day dosing and can be taken either with a meal or on an empty stomach, it is more convenient for patients than zafirlukast, which is a twice-a-day medication and is best taken on an empty stomach. The leukotriene modifiers appear to be most useful in persons with a dual diagnosis of asthma and allergy, especially if allergic rhinitis and asthma co-exist. Leukotriene modifiers are also effective in exercise-induced bronchospasm (EIB), which is described in Question 36.

Rhinitis

An inflammation involving the mucous membranes of the nose. Rhinitis may be allergic or nonallergic.

Long-term control medication must be taken as prescribed, day in and day out, even if symptoms are quiescent. Most controller medications can be left at home and are taken once or twice daily, depending on the medicine and the prescription.

Several years ago, I was completing my pulmonary fellowship at Bellevue Hospital in New York City. An elderly lady with complicated asthma was assigned to my clinic for her care. At first, she had difficulty understanding how and when to use her inhalers. We reviewed the different medicines, which ones were as-needed, quick-relief and which ones were day-in and day-out controllers for maintenance. After a few moments, a broad, triumphant grin spread across my patient's face. "I got it!" she exclaimed. A minute later, she elaborated, "The white inhaler is like my husband—he's always there, morning and night; but, the yellow one is like my boyfriend—he comes around only when I need him!" From that day on, there was no more confusion about those inhalers!

55. Will I need to take asthma medicine forever?

Asthma is characterized by periods of increased activity and of symptom remission, as explained in Question 12. When your asthma is active (persistent, as per the NAEPP classification), you will need to use your asthma medication daily and continue to use it for some time after your asthma becomes better controlled, at which time you may find yourself taking medicine although you feel great! If your asthma becomes quiescent, then you may not need to take daily medicine. That would be the case, if over the last 3 months (or more), you experienced no nocturnal awakenings, no interference with normal activities, and a minimal (or no) need for your inhaled, short-acting, quick-relief β_2 bronchodilator (SABA).

No physician can predict whether or not treatment of your asthma will require indefinite ("forever") medication. I counsel my patients to focus instead on the here and now, addressing right now symptoms rather than becoming caught up in a what-if mentality. The key point is that asthma medicines are highly effective and should be prescribed when necessary. It is wrong to decline appropriate treatment because of a fear of how long that treatment might take!

Medicine is indicated, in the context of an asthma treatment plan, to eliminate respiratory symptoms such as breathlessness, chest discomfort and tightness, cough, wheeze, and exercise limitation. Asthma medicine helps control asthma symptoms, and in doing so clearly improves day-to-day quality of life. Successful asthma management not only includes prescribing the least amount of medicine required for adequate asthma control, but also mandates using medication that is well tolerated and free from undesirable or adverse effects. A basic principle of modern asthma care includes the stepping up and stepping down of medication, reflecting the variable nature of the disease itself and an individual's responsiveness to treatment.

Asthma medicine should always be stepped up until all symptoms become controlled. Current asthma guidelines define six treatment steps in asthma management. Asthma assessments can be obtained as often as weekly if necessary and should focus on the frequency and intensity of lung symptoms and of nocturnal awakenings; the need for inhaled, short-acting, β_2 bronchodilators; any functional limitations; and lung function measurements. The decision to increase the amount of prescribed asthma medicine is thus the result of an ongoing reevaluation targeting the adequacy and maintenance of control. If asthma symptoms are well controlled for at least 90 days in a row, then confirmatory lung function measurements (FEV_1) should be considered along with a clinical assessment, and if control is indeed well established, then asthma medication can be reduced, or "stepped down." It goes without saying that patient and doctor should monitor asthma symptoms closely after a step-down to ensure continued control. If control is maintained, step-down can proceed until minimal or no medication is required.

56. What is the difference between a medicine's generic and brand name?

All medicines will have at least four different names as they make it from the laboratory to your medicine cabinet. When a drug is first developed, it is given a chemical name that describes its molecular composition. Chemical names are accurate descriptors but are complicated and cumbersome, with parentheses and subscripts, numbers and initials. The pharmaceutical company working to develop the drug for market usually will thus give the drug an in-house or code name. The name usually includes letters abbreviating the company's name (for example, or GSK for GlaxoSmithKline), followed by a number. After approval by the U.S. Food and Drug Administration (FDA), the ready-for-market medication is given both a generic and a trade name. Each generic and trade name must be unique and distinctive enough to avoid confusion with other products. In the United States, the United States Adopted Names Council assigns a drug its generic or nonproprietary adopted name. Outside of the United States, the World Health Organization is responsible for a drug's generic international nonproprietary name. The generic name for a widely prescribed, quick-relief, short-acting, inhaled β_2 agonist medicine, for instance, is albuterol in the United States and salbutamol internationally. A medicine's generic name is also its official name. The drug's manufacturer then selects the medicine's trade (or brand) name. The FDA must approve the trade name selected by the manufacturer. To use our previous example, the albuterol sulfate inhaler manufactured by the Schering Company is named Proventil HFA, whereas the inhaler produced by Glaxo-SmithKline is Ventolin HFA. Trade names are often selected to be catchy and easily remembered. The trade name may also reflect a characteristic of the medicine. Many respiratory medicines incorporate *air* or *vent* (as in *ventilation*) as part of the trade name. Examples include Singulair, Advair, Aerobid, Maxair, ProAir, Xolair, Flovent, Serevent, Atrovent, Combivent, Ventolin HFA, and Proventil HFA.

When a new medicine is developed, its inventor applies for a patent for the discovery. The patent details the discovery and, in doing so, makes it public and open to all (including competitors) while protecting the inventor's right to make, use, or sell the medicine for a defined period of time, after which the patent expires. When a medicine is new on the market and its manufacturer is the only producer of that medicine, only one form of the drug is available to the consumer. Eventually, however, the patent protection expires, and other companies may choose to produce the generic form of the medicine. In most cases, the generic form of a medication sold in the United States is pharmacologically equivalent to the brand formulation. Most generic medicine sold in the United States generally costs less than the brand-name medicine and is of good quality; ordinarily, a pharmacist must provide a generic version of a drug unless the physician specifies otherwise. In the state of New York, for example, the pharmacist will dispense a generic formulation of the medication I prescribe for my patients unless I specify "DAW (dispense as written)" on the prescription. Similarly, your physician will have under most circumstances to approve that a prescription medicine be filled with a specific brand rather than a generic formulation.

It is easy to become confused by the fact that a medicine will be called by different names. I always ask my patients to bring all their medicines with them to the office so that we can make sure they understand what medicines they should take and how to take them. I have frequently encountered patients who think that they are taking "a lot of medicine," only to discover that the two separate inhalers they are using are different only because two different manufacturers are producing the same medicine. If a patient is using inhaled Proventil HFA along with inhaled Ventolin HFA, for example, he is really only using one type of drug: albuterol sulfate. Remember that the generic name of a medicine refers to the drug itself, whereas the trade name refers to a specific company's product and brand. For example, aspirin is a generic product; Bufferin is not.

To find out the names of your medicines, ask the doctor or pharmacist, and read labels and package inserts. If you have been prescribed any of the inhaler medications, the label will always carry the drug's trade name along with its generic name, although the generic name will usually be in smaller print. Over-the-counter medicines are also carefully labeled to specify generic and trade names. A trade name on the label is always followed by the ® or ™ symbol, whereas the generic name is not.

Remember that the generic name of a medicine refers to the drug itself, whereas the trade name refers to a specific company's product and brand.

57. Why do I wake up around 2 AM to use my inhaler before going back to sleep?

If you are awakened from sleep in the early morning hours, at 2 or 3 AM for example, with uncomfortable breathing or respiratory symptoms, you are experiencing what asthma specialists refer to as "nocturnal awakenings," or "nocturnal symptoms." Nocturnal awakenings due to asthma are never normal and are undesirable from many points of view. Apart from interfering with sleep and rest, they indicate that your asthma is not adequately controlled and that your asthma is becoming more active. Nocturnal awakenings should always be reported to your treating physician. In the NAEPP classification, a person whose asthma is well controlled experiences nighttime awakenings no more frequently than once a month. If a person with asthma develops nocturnal symptoms more than once a month, the asthma is considered to be persistent and thus by definition, not sufficiently controlled.

Nocturnal awakenings due to asthma are never normal and should always be reported to your treating physician.

When you awaken with asthma symptoms, it is a good idea to use your quick-relief, short-acting, inhaled β_2 (SABA) bronchodilator. It will begin to work within minutes as your asthma symptoms lessen and respond, allowing you to go back to sleep. When you wake up in the morning, you need to give some thought to your asthma. If your asthma was previously under good control, try to figure out why you have developed nocturnal symptoms. Did you omit (or simply forget) your usual asthma medicine? What was your last peak flow (PEF) measurement? Have you been exposed to any known triggers? Did you eat a large, heavy meal right before bedtime, with consequent acid reflux? Are you becoming ill with a viral cold or sinus symptoms? Are your spring allergies flaring?

If you have experienced more than two nighttime asthma episodes in the last 30 days, you probably require additional asthma medicine to regain control of your disease and to prevent an exacerbation. Stepped-up anti-inflammatory and bronchodilator medicine should be considered, and any coincident factors, such as reflux, infection, or allergy, should also be addressed. Remember, a major goal of asthma treatment includes restful, uninterrupted sleep.

Remember, a major goal of asthma treatment includes restful, uninterrupted sleep.

58. Why are so many asthma medicines in inhaler form?

The inhaled route of medication delivery represents an ideal method of treating asthma. Asthma is a disease that involves the lungs and bronchial passageways. It therefore makes perfect sense to deliver the medicine directly where it is needed—right into the air passages. When inhaled correctly, asthma medication goes precisely where it is required, with minimal, if any, absorption by other organs. By limiting the presence of medicine in the bloodstream and other organs, potential drug interactions are avoided and side effects and toxicity are minimized. There are two types of inhalers: metered-dose inhalers (MDIs) and dry-powder inhalers (DPIs). MDIs and DPIs are practical, portable, and fit in a schoolbag, pocket, or handbag. They work at room temperature and can be taken without regard to meals or time of day. With proper instruction, motivated children as young as 5 or 6 years can learn to use inhaled asthma medications, via either an MDI or a DPI. The use of a spacer device such as a holding chamber (reviewed in more detail in Question 66) in combination with an MDI is recommended for all children (and for many adults too) in order to maximize the effectiveness of their MDIs. A listing of available medications used in asthma treatment in inhaler form is presented in Table 37.

59. What is the 1987 Montreal Protocol and why is it relevant to asthma?

The Montreal Protocol is a landmark, international treaty designed to enhance air quality and to protect the uppermost (or stratospheric) ozone layer. In 1987, 24 countries, as well as the European Economic Community, negotiated and signed The Montreal Protocol on Substances that Deplete the Ozone Layer. The initial protocol aimed to decrease the use of ozone-depleting, man-made chemicals by 50% by the year 1999. Additional supplements to the Montreal Protocol, known as the London, Copenhagen, and Beijing Amendments, were adopted in 1990, 1992, and 1999, respectively, and further addressed the use and production of various ozone-depleting chemicals, as well as a timetable for their phaseout.

Ozone is a molecule made up of three oxygen atoms and is an essential constituent of our atmosphere. About 90% of the ozone resides in a layer between 6 and 25 miles above the earth's surface in a zone called the stratosphere. The presence of the correct amount of ozone in the earth's stratosphere is crucial for absorbing dangerous radiation emanating from the sun. The stratosphere's ozone envelops our planet in a kind of protective envelope. For example, increased exposure to the sun's ultraviolet rays, as would occur from depletion of the earth's protective ozone layer, is associated with an increased risk of developing skin cancer and ocular cataracts in humans. Ozone depletion may also adversely affect animal and plant life.

Studies over the last 30 years have revealed a significant decline in the earth's protective ozone layer over Antarctica. The first report of holes in the stratospheric ozone layer by British scientists in May 1985 has been subsequently confirmed and detailed. A widely used class of synthetic chemicals called chlorofluorocarbons (CFCs) has been implicated as a major source of atmospheric ozone depletion. CFCs contain chlorine, fluorine, and carbon atoms. CFCs were invented in the 1920s, and are, in many ways, ideal compounds. CFCs are nontoxic, noncorrosive, and nonflammable. They are inert and nonreactive with most

Chlorofluorocarbons (CFCs)

Chemical propellants previously used in the manufacture of metered-dose inhalers.

substances. In the second half of the 20th century, CFCs found extensive use as propellants in aerosols and spray cans, as coolants in refrigerators and air conditioners, as solvents in cleaners—particularly for electronic circuit boards—and as a blowing agent in the production of foam in devices such as fire extinguishers. Freon, for example, is a familiar brand of a class of CFCs that was used in refrigeration. CFCs are very stable, and it is now recognized that they can persist in the atmosphere for up to 100 years. Any CFC released into the air rises. When CFCs reach the stratosphere, sunlight causes them to break down and release atomic chlorine. The chlorine derived from the CFC is responsible for damaging the ozone layer. Even though the production and release of CFCs have been greatly curtailed, the damage to the ozone layer from past use will continue well into the current century.

The Montreal Protocol was codified by Congress into law in Title VI of the Clean Air Act and stipulated that the production of CFCs in the United States would be banned as of January 1, 1996. Existing medical products that contained CFCs were exempt from the ban until acceptable alternatives could be developed. An essential medical use of CFCs especially relevant to persons with lung disease is the use of CFCs as a propellant in MDIs. MDIs are used extensively in the treatment of asthma, emphysema, and chronic obstructive bronchitis. Although CFCs were no longer used in the manufacture of aerosol spray cans, air conditioners, or refrigeration units after January 1996, they were still produced for pharmaceutical use in some MDIs. Because MDIs are essential for asthma treatment, the Environmental Protection Agency (EPA) and the U.S. Food and Drug Administration (FDA) extended the timeline banning CFC manufacture, and proposed and oversaw the gradual phaseout of all MDIs containing CFCs (MDI-CFC). No CFC-containing

MDIs were removed from the market until safe and effective equivalent medicines became available. A complete ban on the production and sale of single-ingredient albuterol inhalers containing CFCs went into effect in the United States on December 31, 2008, as part of the planet-wide CFC phaseout. Several inhalers in the marketplace now offer CFC-free alternatives.

Pharmaceutical manufacturers have either reformulated their MDI propellants to be CFC free or developed inhaled drug-delivery systems that do not require any propellant at all. Reformulated albuterol MDIs substitute a different, non-CFC type of propellant called hydrofluoroalkane (HFA). The FDA has approved HFA CFC-free MDIs for albuterol, levalbuterol, beclomethasone, fluticasone, and combinations of fluticasone/salmeterol and budesonide/formoterol. The products include ProAir, Proventil HFA, Ventolin HFA, Xopenex, Qvar, MDI Advair, and MDI Symbicort. Other CFC-free products are available in Europe but are not currently approved by the FDA for use in the United States. In addition to producing HFA-propelled MDIs, pharmaceutical manufacturers have devised novel inhalers that do not rely on any propellant whatsoever. Several different controller asthma medicines are now available as DPIs in the United States, and more are sure to follow.

The actual medicine in your current HFA inhaler is identical to that found in your older inhaler.

60. What makes HFA inhaler medicine different from the inhaler medicine I was prescribed a few years ago?

All MDIs contain active asthma medicine along with an inert material called a propellant. The actual medicine in your current HFA inhaler is identical to that found in your older inhaler. The difference lies in an inactive ingredient, the propellant, which as its name indicates, helps to propel the asthma medicine out of the canister. The major determinant of how deeply and effectively the medication enters the breathing passages is, however, up to you. Correct inhalation technique, not the propellant, is responsible for getting the medicine to where it is most effective! The propellant is a substance called a hydrofluoroalkane, abbreviated HFA. As noted in Question 59, the propellant used in most MDIs until recently was a chlorofluorocarbon (CFC), a substance that has been discovered to play a key role in damaging the protective ozone layer of the atmosphere. When it comes to inhaled medications, HFA was deemed the best choice to replace CFC. The reformulation of the propellant used in MDIs does not reduce the effectiveness of your inhaled medication. Studies show that albuterol MDIs with HFA are comparable to CFC MDIs; effectiveness and safety profiles are similar. Interestingly, in the case of the inhaled corticosteroid beclomethasone, the change from CFC to HFA propellant leads to increased amounts of medicine being delivered deeper into the lung, reaching the smallest air passageways, a phenomenon that improves drug delivery and that requires a dose reduction when transitioning from CFC beclomethasone to HFA beclomethasone.

If, for example, you are taking the Ventolin HFA brand of albuterol manufactured by GlaxoSmithKline, you will notice that in addition to the trade name, Ventolin, the label also reads HFA. The active asthma medicine albuterol (a short-acting, quick-relief β_2 agonist) in the newer HFA inhaler is identical to the albuterol in the older CFC inhaler; only the propellant is different. The medicine is the same, carries the same name, works just as effectively, and has the added benefit of including a dose counter. The labeling of newer inhalers is more accurate because it specifies which inert propellant (HFA) is used in your MDI. The change to an HFA inhaler, however, means that you must learn new inhaler facts, as outlined in Table 39.

All HFA inhalers require priming prior to first use. That means that you must release a specified number of puffs into the air before you then inhale your first dose from a new MDI or from one that you have not used for some time. Be sure to familiarize yourself with the manufacturer's instructions (available from your pharmacist or online) so that you know if your inhaler requires three or four priming puffs. Proventil HFA, Ventolin HFA, and Xopenex HFA require four sprays to prime the inhaler, whereas ProAir requires three sprays. HFA inhalers require repriming sprays if they are not used regularly. Some inhalers may require such a repriming if 2 or more days have elapsed; be certain you know the specifics as they apply to the medicine you have been prescribed! Another fact is that all HFA inhalers have a shelf life; they will need to be discarded after you have released the number of puffs contained in the canister or after a certain amount of time has

HFA inhalers require repriming sprays if they are not used regularly.

Table 39 Facts About Hydrofluoroalkane (HFA) Containing Inhalers

- HFA replaced CFC in albuterol containing metered-dose inhalers in the United States as of January 1, 2009.
- HFA is contained in quick-relief, rapid acting albuterol metered dose inhalers.
- HFA is contained in some long-acting (LABA) daily-use inhaled β_2 bronchodilators.
- HFA is contained in some daily-use inhaled corticosteroid (ICS) inhalers.
- HFA, like CFC, is an inert propellant and is not an asthma medicine.
- HFA containing metered-dose inhalers as compared to CFC containing metered-dose inhalers:
  - Contain the same *active* asthma medication as CFC inhalers
  - Have different priming instructions/requirements than CFC inhalers
  - Need to be cleaned more frequently than CFC inhalers
  - Create a "softer" spray of medicine than CFC inhalers
  - Do not contribute to depletion of the stratosphere's ozone layer: "greener"

passed since you first removed the inhaler from its protective overwrap. If your HFA MDI has an incorporated dose counter (such as Ventolin HFA), you will know exactly how many doses remain before you will need to refill your prescription. If your inhaler does not have a dose counter, then you must keep track of how many doses you have used up so that you can calculate how many doses remain in the canister. Note that the quick-relief, inhaled, short-acting β_2 (SABA) bronchodilators containing albuterol, ProAir, Proventil HFA, Ventolin HFA, or Xopenex HFA all contain 200 doses per canister. All HFA MDIs are adversely affected by moisture and so are packaged in a protective overwrap after they are manufactured. Once the wrap is opened, the MDI becomes exposed to air and the medicine must be used or discarded within a relatively short period. Each medicine is different; some must be replaced as soon as 60 days after opening, so make certain you find out what applies in the case of the medicine that you have been prescribed. There is obviously no point inhaling from an MDI if there is no active medicine available to benefit you!

HFA inhalers have a gentler, weaker spray and require generation of a slower inhalation compared to the older CFC inhalers; you will not "feel" a spray of HFA in the same manner you did when using a CFC inhaler. HFA inhalers also create a warmer spray compared to the older CFC inhalers, and you may notice a distinct taste. Because HFA is stickier than CFC, the mouthpiece will require weekly rinsing to prevent clogging the inhaler hole (Table 40). The American College of Chest Physicians advises that "The mouthpiece should be cleaned once weekly by running warm water through the top and bottom for 30 seconds (remove the metal canister first) and then shaking vigorously to remove excess water. This should be followed by air drying overnight. As with

Table 40   Hydrofluoroalkane (HFA) Containing Inhalers: Experts' View

- Proventil HFA, the first CFC inhaled albuterol, has been in use in the United States for over a decade.
- All HFA inhalers MUST be primed prior to first use. Different brands of medication may require either three or four priming puffs. HFA inhalers require re-priming sprays if not used regularly. Check the manufacturer's specifics. Proventil HFA, Ventolin HFA, and Xopenex HFA require four sprays to prime the inhaler, for instance, whereas ProAir requires three sprays.
- All HFA inhalers require a slower inhalation than older, CFC containing inhalers.
- All HFA inhalers have a gentler, weaker spray as compared to the older CFC inhalers; you will not "feel" a spray of HFA as you would with a CFC inhaler. ProAir has the "softest" spray.
- All HFA inhalers create a warmer spray as compared to the older CFC inhalers.
- HFA is "stickier" than CFC and the mouthpiece of all HFA inhalers requires regular (weekly) rinsing to prevent clogging the inhaler hole.
- *Never* immerse any HFA (or CFC) metal canister in water.
- One HFA inhaler (Ventolin HFA) has an incorporated dose-counter.
- Of the rapid-acting quick-relief inhaled short-acting β_2 (SABA) bronchodilators, ProAir, Proventil HFA, Ventolin HFA, and Xopenex HFA contain 200 doses per canister.
- All HFA inhalers must be discarded after a certain amount of time has elapsed (check the specifics for your medicine) even if not all doses were used.
- No generic HFA inhalers will become available until current patent protections expire. If you are experiencing difficulty paying for your prescriptions, you might consider contacting the Partnership for Prescription Assistance: http://www.pparx.org/ or 1-888-4PPA-NOW (1-888-477-2669) for assistance.
- All HFA inhalers are environmentally friendlier as compared to the older CFC inhalers that contained an ozone-depleting substance.

Source: Adapted from the American College of Chest Physicians http://www.chestnet.org/networks/ airway_disorders/hotTopics.php

CFC-based inhalers, the metal canisters should never be submerged in water or allowed to get wet."

Generic HFA inhalers will not become available until current patent protections expire. HFA inhalers sold in the United States thus cost more than their generic CFC predecessors did. GlaxoSmithKline, the manufacturer of Ventolin HFA that contains 200 puffs (doses) per canister makes an HFA inhaler that contains 60 puffs (doses) called ReliOn Ventolin HFA. ReliOn HFA inhalers are distributed exclusively through Walmart stores. One canister of 60 doses costs less than the standard 200-dose albuterol MDI, so ReliOn Ventolin might be an option if you use albuterol infrequently. In general, if you are experiencing difficulty paying for your prescriptions, you should let your treating doctor know of your circumstances, and you might also consider contacting the Partnership for Prescription Assistance: http://www.pparx.org/ or 1-888-4PPA-NOW (1-888-477-2669).

61. What is a Diskus? Is it the same as a DPI?

Yes, the Diskus is one type of DPI device used in asthma treatment. Other DPI devices that allow for inhalation of asthma medicines include the Aerolizer, the Flexhaler (previously called the Turbuhaler), and the Twisthaler. Some devices such as the Diskhaler and the Clickhaler are not available in the United States but are used abroad.

DPIs are devices that permit a person with asthma to self-administer precise, predetermined doses of inhaled corticosteroids or long-acting bronchodilator medicine, either individually or in combination. DPIs were developed as an alternative delivery device to CFC-containing MDIs. From a technical point of view, patients usually find it easier to use a DPI than an MDI. Using a DPI requires you to take a controlled, deep breath from the DPI mouthpiece in such a manner that the medication, which is in the form of a very fine powder, penetrates deeply into the bronchial passageways. Although DPIs and MDIs both dispense very precise doses of medication, DPIs are fundamentally different from MDIs. The DPI device automatically releases medicine as you generate an inward flow of air with your lips around the

Dry-powder inhaler (DPI)

A newer method of delivering medication directly to the lungs and respiratory passages. DPIs are supplanting traditional MDIs partly because of their ease of use, convenience, and good patient acceptance.

mouthpiece. The DPI is thus breath activated or patient activated; it requires less coordination compared to an MDI. You must be able to generate sufficient airflow through the mouthpiece in order to benefit from a dry-powder inhaler. As a rule, DPIs can be prescribed for persons over 5 years of age, as younger children do not have the ability to generate the required airflow to trigger the release of medicine from the device.

One type of DPI (such as the Diskus, the Twisthaler, and the Flexhaler) has a month's supply of asthma medicine already contained in the device. You bring up each dose, as it is needed, usually by clicking a lever or by rotating the base of the DPI unit immediately before use. The second type of DPI requires that you open the DPI before the time of use and place a capsule that contains a single dose of medicine in powdered form into a groove or chamber before snapping the DPI back into place. Medicines provided through the Diskus, the Flexhaler (previously known as a Turbuhaler), and the Twisthaler are preloaded with a month's supply of medicine. The Aerolizer requires that you place a capsule containing the medicine into the device right before each use. A Handihaler similarly needs to be loaded immediately prior to each dose, but it delivers a medication (tiotropium) that is currently FDA approved for the treatment of lung conditions other than asthma (COPD and emphysema).

The design of the Diskus is distinctive—it looks like a small disc—and features a small counter that displays how many doses remain in the device, which is a very useful and practical feature. The Flexhaler and Twisthaler have a more tubelike shape and have incorporated dose counters as well, to let you know when it is time to obtain a refill from the pharmacy. Several different types of asthma medicines come in DPI form, including long-acting β_2 agonists (LABAs such as sal-meterol and formoterol), inhaled corticosteroids (such as budesonide, fluticasone, and mometasone), and combi-nation DPIs containing different potency inhaled corti-costeroids, directly combined with long-acting β_2 agonists (such as mixtures of salmeterol with fluticasone and, outside of the United States, budesonide with formoterol DPI). Trade names include the Serevent Diskus, Foradil Aerolizer, Pulmicort Flexhaler, Flovent Diskus, Flovent Rotadisk Diskhaler, Asmanex Twisthaler, and Advair Diskus.

62. What is the correct way to use my DPI?

DPIs deliver asthma medicine as very fine particles of powder. As discussed in Question 61, there are many types of DPIs available on the market in the United States. Additional DPIs are sold abroad. Each type of DPI is manufactured by a different pharmaceutical company, and each type of DPI consequently has its specific set of instructions for optimal use. When your physician prescribes a DPI for treatment of your asthma, have him or her demonstrate the correct way for you to use the DPI and provide you with any avail-able instructional materials. When you fill the pre-scription, make sure that the dispensing pharmacist includes the directions provided by the manufacturer. Some pharmacists can advise you on proper DPI usage techniques. Finally, instructions and video demonstrations are available on the Internet on both pharmaceutical and medical Web sites. You can easily access a manufacturer's Web site by typing your med-icine's name into a search engine's search box. Web sites not maintained by pharmaceutical companies are other resources you may wish to consult to learn more about your specific inhaled medicine. The Mayo Clinic's Web site is an example of a medical site that includes links to videos showing how to use a disk inhaler (like the Diskus) as well as a tube inhaler (like the Flexhaler or Twisthaler). You can see them at www.mayoclinic.com/health/asthma/MM00405 and www.mayoclinic.com/health/asthma/MM00404, respectively. Another excellent resource is the Web site maintained by National Jewish Health, a hospital system dedicated to lung disease and respiratory health. It has detailed information with videos on all the different DPIs at www.nationaljewish.org/healthinfo/medications/lung-diseases/devices/dry-powder/index.aspx.

Even though each DPI comes with its own set of instructions, all DPIs share similar conceptual and design features. They are prized for their ease of use, reliability, efficiency, and convenience. All DPIs are breath activated. When you inhale through a DPI, a precisely premeasured dose of medicine is automatically released. The way you breathe the medicine in (your inhaler technique) allows the drug to travel into your airways where it is needed. The general principle is that you should inhale the medicine via the DPI mouthpiece starting with empty lungs and then hold your breath before exhaling and breathing normally. The basic technique consists of an initial exhalation to empty your lungs, followed by a steady, fairly rapid inhalation from the mouthpiece, and breath holding.

To use a DPI correctly, you first prepare the premeasured dose of medicine, either by rotating and clicking the base of a tube shaped device, advancing a small lever on a disk-shaped inhaler, or by physically inserting powder-containing capsules into a specially designed groove in the device, depending on which type of DPI you have been prescribed. When the medicine is ready, you take in a big breath of room air and then fully exhale it into the room. Once your lungs are completely empty, place your lips around the DPI's mouthpiece and steadily take a full, deep breath, inhaling the medicine until you cannot breathe in any further. You should not "taste" or "feel" the inhaled medicine. Once you reach the point when your lungs are full of medicine, hold your breath. You should attempt to hold your breath for up to 10 seconds before exhaling. Count to 10 in your head. After you reach a count of 10, remove the DPI mouthpiece from your lips, and let your breath out. Remember to exhale into the room. Do not exhale into a DPI device.

The reason you need to hold your breath after taking the inhaled dose of medicine is to allow the medicine to deposit in the air passages. When you hold your breath, there is no movement of air in the lungs. Since there is no flow of air, either in or out, your asthma medicine remains in the lungs long enough to be of benefit to you.

The reason you need to hold your breath after taking the inhaled dose of medicine is to allow the medicine to deposit in the air passages.

Become familiar with the specific DPI device you have been prescribed. Read the manufacturer's instructions for patient use insert provided with the product. Ask your treating physician any questions you may have. I often ask my patients to bring their DPI with them to their appointment so that they can demonstrate how they use it. I am then able to assess the effectiveness of their technique and, if appropriate, make specific suggestions for improvement. Note that each DPI not only looks unique, but also has specific characteristics. For example, the disposable Diskus device is packaged in a foil pouch, and its manufacturer states that a Diskus should be used or discarded within 1 month of opening the foil pouch to prevent the medicine from drying out. A Twisthaler must be discarded 45 days after opening or when the counter reads a zero, whichever occurs first. The Diskus and the Twisthaler also have incorporated dosage counters that indicate how many doses of medicine remain in the device. When the 0 is displayed, your DPI is empty. You should always keep a DPI inhaler in horizontal position when you place your lips around the mouthpiece to inhale medicine. If you are left-handed, you may find it more comfortable and natural to turn the Diskus device over and use it with the label facing down, so that the lever is easier to click into position with your left thumb while holding the device in your left hand. The Diskus should be closed to cover the mouthpiece after each use and does not require any other maintenance or cleaning. To avoid introducing moisture into a DPI, never exhale into the device.

The Flexhaler is similar to the Diskus in that it comes preloaded with medicine. It is shaped like a tube. In order for you to prepare your dose of medicine, the Flexhaler requires you to twist the brown grip at the base of the device fully in one direction as far as it will go and then twist it fully back again in the other direction before you place the mouthpiece between your lips and inhale after a deep exhalation as described above. It does not matter which way you turn first, clockwise or counterclockwise. You will hear a confirmatory click as you twist. The Flexhaler needs to be primed before you first use it; and as is the case with all DPIs, you should never exhale into the device mouthpiece, which will introduce moisture into the device. The Flexhaler has a dose counter window below the mouthpiece. It does not actually display the exact amount of doses remaining in the device, but will let you know approximately how many doses are left. As you use the Flexhaler, the numbers will count down by 10. The Flexhaler will count down to 0, which will appear in the center of the window when the Flexhaler is empty. Plan to get a new Flexhaler before you see the 0 in the window. Always recap the Flexhaler after using it to keep it clean and dry; you can wipe the mouthpiece with a dry cloth, but do not wash the device.

Another tube-shaped DPI is the Twisthaler. It has a pink colored base (in contrast to the brown Flexhaler's base) and has a dose counter that counts down how many doses remain in the device. As the case for the Flexhaler, you will need to prepare the dose by holding the Twisthaler upright and twisting the white cap counterclockwise, which puts the medicine in the device. Once the medicine is good to go, you can empty your lungs of air and inhale your medicine, as described earlier in this section.

The Aerolizer and Handihaler devices require that you load capsules that contain medicine into the DPI before use, and they accept only one dose at a time.

63. What is the correct way to use my MDI?

MDIs are convenient, portable, and highly reliable devices designed to deliver active medicine directly into the lungs by inhalation. MDIs are conceptually similar to DPIs (discussed in Questions 61 and 62). Both MDIs and DPIs allow for the delivery of accurate, pre-determined doses of medicine directly to the respiratory passages. MDIs and DPIs also exhibit fundamental differences. All MDIs use a propellant to push the medicine out of its dosing canister. Except for the Maxair Autohaler, the MDIs on the market in the United States are manually activated rather than breath activated. Manually activated means that the medicine is released

Metered-dose inhalers (MDIs) are convenient, portable, and highly reliable devices designed to deliver active medicine directly into the lungs by inhalation.

from the MDI canister when you press down on (or actuate) the MDI. Breath activated means that the medicine is automatically released when you inhale deeply; the inward flow of air as you inhale triggers the medication release. Because most MDIs are manually activated, their proper use is technically more demanding and requires more coaching and more learning at the onset, as compared with DPIs.

The correct way to use your MDI is best demonstrated by your physician. There are two techniques for best use: the open-mouth and the closed-mouth technique. All MDIs come with directions. The directions on the manufacturer's package insert describe the closed-mouth technique. Pulmonary specialists (such as me) generally prefer to teach their patients the open-mouth method of using the MDI. Many pulmonary specialists believe that using the MDI with an open mouth enhances the delivery of medicine and favors the inhalation of the more desirable, smaller particles released by the MDI. You can read detailed information about each technique on the American College of Chest Physicians (ACCP) patient information pages, *Using Inhaled Devices,* online at http://www.chestnet.org/accp/patient-guides/patient-instructions-inhaled-devices-english-and-spanish.

MDIs should be stored at room temperature, between 68°F and 77°F (20°C–25°C). Avoid subjecting any MDI to sustained temperatures below 59°F or above 77°F. MDIs should be stored in a vertical position (upright, not on its side) with the mouthpiece down when not in use. If you notice that the plastic mouthpiece becomes coated with a whitish powder, pull the metal MDI canister out from the plastic mouthpiece and clean the mouthpiece. Each MDI manufacturer has specific instructions on how to clean the mouthpiece, so be sure to check the correct method for the medicine you have been prescribed. All newer HFA MDI mouthpieces require once a week maintenance cleaning as per the manufacturer's instructions. Always make sure the mouthpiece is completely dry before reinserting the metal canister. It is fine to let the plastic part air-dry.

All MDIs should be allowed to reach room temperature before use. If you carry your quick-relief MDI with you, and you are outdoors on an especially cold day, place it in an inner pocket close to your body rather than in a handbag or backpack. Never leave an MDI in the glove compartment or in the trunk of your car on a hot day; its contents are under pressure and can explode in very hot environments (120°F or above). Several years ago, one of my patients didn't seem to be faring as well as I had expected. She was an elderly widow and lived alone. She and I spent an entire office visit carefully going over what had changed to explain her loss of asthma control. Imagine my consternation when she confided that she had hit on a great way to remember where she had put her MDIs: She stored them in her refrigerator's vegetable drawer, at around 40°F. She would take them from the vegetable bin, and go through the process of using the MDI, not realizing that they needed to be stored in a warmer environment, and certainly warmed to room temperature before use! After we decided that she should keep her medicines on the top of the chest of drawers in the bedroom, her asthma once again became controlled, to our mutual satisfaction.

The general concept in using an MDI is that you trigger the release of medicine from the MDI while simultaneously inhaling the medication into empty lungs. The basic technique consists of an initial exhalation to empty your lungs, release of a puff of medication to coincide with a full, steady, deep inhalation, followed by breath holding.

To use your MDI, first remove the cap from the mouthpiece. Ideally, you should stand to use your inhaler. If you prefer to be seated, make sure that you sit upright. Hold the inhaler upright, with the mouthpiece at the bottom. Many people find it most comfortable to hold the MDI with their thumb at the lowermost portion and their third finger on the topmost metal portion of the MDI canister. Next, shake the MDI canister to mix the medicine. After shaking the MDI, position the mouthpiece 2 to 3 finger widths (1 to 2 in.) in front of your open mouth. Tilt your head back slightly, and gently breathe out. When you have emptied your lungs, press on the MDI and simultaneously take a slow, deep breath. Keep inhaling for at least 5 seconds. Once you have inhaled fully, hold your breath to allow the medicine to fully penetrate in your lungs and deposit there. Try to hold your breath for 10 seconds. Exhale and resume normal breathing. If your doctor has prescribed a second puff of medication, you may be instructed to wait a minute or more between doses. The MDI-delivered medicine should be going straight into your lungs; consequently, it not should irritate your throat or cause you to cough, nor should it land on your tongue or have any taste. It is important that you learn to use your prescribed MDI correctly. Make sure you ask your physician any questions you may have about the way you are using your MDI (Table 41). I have found it very useful to watch my patients' MDI technique during an office visit. A well-worded or carefully-timed pointer can make a world of difference. Remember that mastering good MDI technique involves a learning curve, and with proper instruction and supervision, even young children can use MDI-delivered asthma medication.

Remember that mastering good MDI technique involves a learning curve, and with proper instruction and supervision, even young children can use MDI-delivered asthma medication.

Table 41   Metered Dose Inhalers: Common Errors in Technique

- Forgetting to shake the MDI before use
- Not priming the MDI before use, in accordance with the specific instructions of the manufacturer
- Sitting in a hunched over position when inhaling from your MDI
- Blocking the MDI opening with your tongue or teeth
- Releasing the puff of medicine either before ("too soon") or after ("too late") you have initiated a deep breath ("poor coordination pattern")
- Taking in too shallow a breath
- Not holding your breath for at least 10 seconds after inhaling your medicine
- Neglecting to rinse your mouth ("rinse & spit") after using your inhaled corticosteroid MDI
- Forgetting to discard the MDI when no doses of medicine remain in the canister
- Forgetting to learn for how many months you can use an MDI dispensed in a moisture-proof foil before it must be discarded (even if there is still medicine inside)

64. Why does my doctor say I should rinse my mouth after using my MDI?

Your doctor has instructed you to rinse your mouth after using your inhaler in order to gently wash away any medicine particles that were not inhaled into the lungs and may have remained behind in your throat. It is especially important to rinse your mouth after each use of any of the daily-use maintenance anti-inflammatory inhaled corticosteroid (ICS) preparations, whether administered by MDI, DPI, or nebulizer. The inhaled corticosteroid medications can, if they land in your throat, cause some throat irritation, and occasionally lead to a yeast infection in the mouth or throat called thrush. Rinsing your mouth and gargling is thought to reduce your chances of getting thrush and decreases the chance that you will experience throat irritation or hoarseness. Remember to rinse and then spit; do not swallow the liquid you gargled with!

65. How can I tell when my inhaler is empty?

It is easy to know when a DPI is empty because DPIs have incorporated dose counters that help you keep track of how many doses remain in the inhaler and remind you when to refill your prescription. Some dose counters count down as you use each dose or puff of medicine. Others count down every 10 doses. The Diskus device counts down each time you inhale a dose, and when five doses remain in the DPI, a red number 5 appears in the window, followed by a red 4, 3, 2, 1, and then 0. The Twisthaler device also counts down for you until "00" appears in the display. The Flexhaler counts down by ten—the display will not change after each puff—until zero is reached. It is a good idea to keep an eye on how many doses remain in your DPI so that you can refill your prescription before you run out of medicine. Never use a DPI when the dose counter reads zero. Preloaded DPIs are dispensed by your pharmacist in a moisture-protective foil wrapper. The instructions for patients that come with the prescribed DPI will specify how long a DPI can be kept before it has to be replaced with fresh medicine. An Advair containing Diskus DPI must be discarded within 30 days of opening the foil wrapper, regardless of whether or not the counter registers 0 doses. A Serevent Diskus DPI must be discarded within 6 weeks of opening the foil wrapper, regardless of how many doses of drug remain in the device. Similarly, Asmanex Twisthaler has to be thrown away after 45 days, even if the counter indicates that a few doses remain in the device.

Four MDIs available in the United States have built-in dose counters. The MDIs with incorporated dose-counters are Advair HFA, Flovent HFA, Symbicort HFA, and Ventolin HFA. The first three medications are daily use, control medicines, and the fourth is a quick-relief, short-acting β_2 agonist bronchodilator. All four have dose counters that count down as you use up the medicine, making it clear when only a few doses remain in the device.

All MDIs contain active medicine and a propellant (HFA) as described in Questions 59 and 60. It is important to understand that once the active medicine has been used up, propellant may remain in the MDI canister. Even though no medicine remains in the device, it is not entirely empty. That is why you cannot tell if an MDI is empty by shaking it. Once you have used the number of medication doses contained in any MDI, you should discard it. If you continue to use that particular MDI (something I obviously discourage) you will be inhaling propellant!

You cannot tell if an MDI is empty by shaking it.

If you have been prescribed Advair HFA, Flovent HFA, Symbicort HFA, or Ventolin HFA, the dose counters will let you know when a canister is out of medicine. If your MDI inhaler does not have an incorporated dose counter, the only way to be certain that an MDI still has medicine in it is to actually count each (and every) dose as you use the medicine. Small, external counters that fit in the palm of your hand can be clicked each time you use the MDI, an accurate but not always convenient solution. External dose counters that attach to MDIs are also on the market. Another option involves estimating ahead of time when you will need to replace the MDI. Your estimate is based on how many doses (or actuations) the MDI contains and how frequently you use the MDI. For example, consider an MDI whose label states that it contains 100 puffs of medicine. If you take one puff of the medication twice daily the new MDI should provide enough medicine for 50 days; dividing 100

Actuation

The action that releases a dose of medication from a metered-dose inhaler (MDI).

(the number of doses in the MDI) by 2 (the number of doses used in 1 day). You can also ask your pulmonary doctor or pharmacist to help you anticipate when you will need to obtain an MDI refill. You divide the total number of doses in the full MDI by the number of daily doses you plan to use to determine for how many days the MDI will last. Consider writing the date in your calendar or PDA ahead of time so you remember to contact your pharmacist a few days ahead of the expected empty MDI date.

Various strategies have been advanced over the years to help you know when your MDI is empty or nearly empty. As noted above, shaking the inhaler is an unreliable method of assessing whether or not the inhaler still contains medication. Another idea that is not recommended involves removing the metal MDI canister from its plastic mouthpiece and dropping the canister into a glass of water to see if it floats near the surface, which would indicate that it is empty or nearly so. MDI manufacturers and the NAEPP are strongly opposed to immersing the metal MDI canister in water, so floating any MDI canister is a no-no under any circumstances. The potency of inhaled medications cannot be guaranteed if the canister is immersed in water.

Finally, note that Ventolin HFA with an incorporated dose counter and Symbicort HFA, a quick-acting, rapid-relief bronchodilator and a daily-use controller medicine respectively, are packaged in moisture-proof protective pouches. Once you open the pouch, each medicine must be used within a specific amount of time to ensure its effectiveness. The Ventolin HFA with an incorporated dose counter must be discarded 6 months after the pouch is opened, even if the dose counter does not yet read "000." Symbicort HFA must be discarded 3 months after opening, even if not all the 120 doses it contains have been all used up.

66. What is a valved holding chamber, and why should I purchase one?

A valved holding chamber (VHC) is a commercially manufactured device that is designed to be used in conjunction with MDIs. VHCs make it easier to inhale asthma medicines from MDIs, increase the amount of medicine delivered directly to the lungs, and reduce potential side effects such as voice hoarseness and thrush. Purchasing a VHC in the United States requires a prescription. Examples of VHCs are the AeroChamber, AeroChamber Max, OptiChamber, ProChamber, and the Pari Vortex. VHCs are recommended for all children with asthma who use MDIs, but VHCs are useful for adults as well.

A valved holding chamber (VHC) is a commercially manufactured device that is designed to be used in conjunction with metered-dose inhalers (MDIs).

Most valved holding chambers are rigid and shaped like a tube, with a mouthpiece (or face mask) on one end and an opening at the other. The end with a mouthpiece is also manufactured with a face mask for use by children under 5 years of age. The opening at the opposite end accepts the mouthpiece of the MDI containing your medicine. The VHC is designed with a one-way valve that allows the actuation (puff) released from the MDI to enter the chamber and from there be inhaled. The one-way valve prevents you from breathing into the device; you can only inhale from it. Of the VHCs mentioned, the AeroChamber, OptiChamber, and ProChamber are made of a transparent plastic material that allows you to actually see the plume of medication as it is released from the MDI. That can be useful if you are helping a child with his or her inhaler since the visual cue may help you with timing as you instruct the youngster to inhale the medicine. The Pari Vortex is a valved holding chamber made of aluminum, which has the advantages of being nonelectrostatic as well as dishwasher safe, although you obviously cannot see the medication as it is released from the MDI. Nonelectrostatic chambers (such as the aluminum Vortex and the AeroChamber Max) have, in laboratory experiments, been shown to absorb less of the medicine, making more drug available for inhalation. The chambers made of plastic require monthly rinsing in diluted dishwasher detergent (1 part detergent to 5,000 parts water, or 1–2 drops per cup of water) followed by air-drying to counteract electrostatic charges (think static cling!) that can interfere with the VHC's effectiveness. Do not rub or towel dry a VHC. Although there are many studies of VHC use with asthma medicines in persons with asthma that show benefit, the latest *Expert Panel Report* (*EPR-3*) points out that "no specific combination of MDI and VHC currently has been specifically approved by the FDA for use together." The EPR further suggests "it may be preferable to use the same combination of MDI and VHC reported" in the published study of a particular asthma medication. Your doctor should be able to advise you on which specific holding chamber is best for the MDI you have been prescribed.

If your treating physician has advised that you use a VHC with your MDI, make sure to read the instructions applicable to the particular VHC that you have purchased. You should understand how to use your VHC and how to clean it. Perhaps your doctor will directly demonstrate how to use the chamber with an MDI. It is also a good idea to bring the device with you to your appointment so that your technique can be observed in action!

VHCs are different from spacers. *Spacers* is a general term used to describe any simple open tube, without a one-way valve, that extends from the mouthpiece of an MDI. Some MDIs are manufactured with incorporated spacers. Azmacort MDI (the brand of triamcinolone manufactured by Kos Pharmaceuticals), a daily-use, maintenance inhaled corticosteroid medication, is an example of a medication furnished with an incorporated spacer. You should always inhale your Azmacort brand of triamcinolone through the spacer that comes with it. Some spacers are homemade devices, such as plastic bottles or cardboard tubes. Some physicians use the terms *spacer* and *valved holding chamber* interchangeably. They are not synonymous, as you now know!

VHCs are different from spacers.

The benefits of using a valved holding chamber are at least threefold (Table 42). The VHC enhances the delivery of the MDI's medication into the lung passages. It reduces potential side effects such as cough, hoarseness, thrush, and throat irritation related to asthma medicine landing in the throat. More medicine goes where it is needed, the lung airways, and less where it is not. VHCs also greatly simplify the hardest step for most MDI users: having to coordinate and precisely time inhalation

Table 42   Valved Holding Chambers

Valved holding chambers (VHCs):
- Are indicated for any person who has difficulty performing adequate MDI technique
- Are advised for children
- Decrease deposition of medicine in the mouth and throat
- Decrease the risk of some side effects, such as hoarseness and thrush
- If not non-electrostatic, must be rinsed monthly with dilute dishwashing detergent and air dried
- Differ from spacers as VHCs have a one-way valve that allows only inhaling from the device
- Are preferred to spacers, which do not contain a one-way valve

with activation and pumping of the canister. You use a valved holding chamber by inserting the mouthpiece of the MDI at the far end of the tube and placing your lips around the VHC's mouthpiece at the opposite end. First, depress the MDI canister to release one (not more!) puff of medicine into the VHC, and then inhale deeply and steadily before holding your breath for 10 seconds or more. Some VHCs make a whistling sound if you breathe in too fast. Learn to inhale so that the spacer remains silent. What is a one-step procedure with MDIs becomes a two-step process with the MDI+VHC combination.

Kerrin's comment:

Now that my son is getting a bit older, his allergy specialist prescribed an albuterol MDI with a holding chamber for him to use when he needs it. The inhaler fits right into one end of the tube, and there is a soft, rubber-rimmed mask that fits over the nose and mouth on the other end. And rather than sitting for 15–20 minutes with the nebulizer, this delivers the medicine in twelve breaths (six breaths for each of two pushes on the MDI canister). It's much more convenient to use because I don't have to look for an electrical socket and a place to sit comfortably for 15–20 minutes with a squirmy child.

Nebulizer

A device that transforms a respiratory drug in liquid form into a fine mist of medicine particles that are easily inhaled into the respiratory passages. It is powered by a machine or compressor that runs off electrical current or batteries.

67. What is a nebulizer, and how do I use one?

A nebulizer is device powered by electrical current or batteries that creates a fine mist of medicine particles that can be inhaled into the lungs' breathing passages. Nebulizers are fitted with either a mouthpiece or a face mask. Babies and very young children are candidates for the latter. Many different medications used in asthma treatment are manufactured in a liquid form suitable for nebulization. The two major types of nebulizers are jet nebulizers and ultrasonic nebulizers. Most pulmonologists prefer jet nebulizers for their patients as they produce more uniformly sized medicine particles for inhalation. If you or your child has been prescribed Pulmicort Respules, which is an inhaled steroid preparation, it must be administered by a jet nebulizer. The Respules should not be given by ultrasonic nebulization.

The machine that transforms the liquid medication into a fine mist is the nebulizer, and the part of the apparatus that permits the mist to be inhaled is the air compressor. All nebulizer units consist of a nebulizer proper as well as a small cup to hold the liquid form of medication. Special tubing connects the nebulizer proper to the air compressor that sends air though the medication cup and transforms the liquid medicine into a fine mist suitable for inhalation. Several studies have revealed that the different nebulizers available on the market have different medication-delivery profiles. Although all nebulizers work in a similar way, you should familiarize yourself fully with the nebulizer that your physician prescribes for you or your child. Read any directions for use and maintenance carefully. Many nebulizer manufacturers maintain Web sites for their products and can be a good source of information for patients.

To use your nebulizer you will need to assemble the nebulizer and air compressor, inhale the nebulized medication (treatment), which should last about 15–20 minutes, clean and prepare the nebulizer for the next use, and every other day, perform a more thorough cleaning.

Here are some general guidelines on how to use your nebulizer, using a mouthpiece. Babies and young children will need to use a special mask rather than a mouthpiece. Understand that your individual machine may require slightly different handling. First, always collect all the equipment and medicine you will require, including the nebulizer, tubing, medicine, and the compressor. Wash your hands. Use a clean nebulizer and fill the medication cup with one dose of your medicine as directed by your physician. Connect the air tubing between the nebulizer and the compressor, along with a finger valve if your setup requires one. Attach a mouthpiece or mask to the nebulizer. Turn the compressor on and check that the nebulizer is producing a medication mist. Now you are ready to place your lips around the mouthpiece. You should stabilize the mouthpiece between your teeth. Remember to hold the nebulizer upright to avoid spills, and to increase its effectiveness. Breathe gently and calmly. Try to breathe in deeply for 3–5 seconds before holding your breath for up to 10 seconds, and then exhale normally. If your nebulizer has a finger valve, you should cover the hole in the finger valve while you inhale, and uncover the valve when you exhale. Repeat, drawing deep breaths, followed by breath holds until the nebulizer begins to make sputtering sounds. The sputtering sound signals that your treatment is finished.

When all the medication solution has been nebulized, take the nebulizer setup apart. Wash all the parts—except for the tubing and the finger valve—in liquid dish soap and water. Rinse in tap water, and shake off any excess water droplets. Reconnect the different parts and run the compressor to dry the nebulizer. Wait until the nebulizer is completely dry before storing it. If you use a nebulizer daily, you should also perform a more in-depth cleaning every 48 hours or so. To do so, wash your hands first. Then, put aside the tubing and valve. Prepare a fresh solution of distilled white vinegar and hot water. The proportions are 1 part white vinegar to 3 parts hot water (one quarter white vinegar to three quarters hot water). Soak all parts of the nebulizer (except the tubing and mask) in the vinegar and hot water solution for 60 minutes. After an hour, remove the nebulizer parts and rinse them under running water. Throw away the soaking solution. After rinsing in fresh water, shake off any excess water droplets. Reconnect the different parts of the setup, and run the compressor to dry the nebulizer. Wait until the nebulizer is completely dry before storing it. Make it a point to find out whether the compressor unit you are using requires additional specific maintenance or cleaning.

Some people use the term *breathing machine* interchangeably with the term *nebulizer*. Strictly speaking, the nebulizer is the device at the end of the tubing from the compressor, and not the entire setup. That said, most people, including doctors, refer to the entire machine—the compressor, tubing, medication cup, and mouthpiece (or face mask)—collectively as "the nebulizer."

Kerrin's comment:

My son was first given his nebulizer when he was about 8 months old. He quickly got used to it and will now ask for a treatment if he's feeling uncomfortable. We have learned that it is a good idea to bring the nebulizer with us (and plenty of albuterol) if we are going to a place where a trigger might be present, such as a friend's house or an outdoor event. We also know it is important to remember to pack it when going on vacation, along with enough medication to last if my son gets a respiratory illness that could potentially trigger symptoms.

68. Is medication in nebulized form more effective than that in an inhaler?

The surprising answer is, "No, not necessarily and not usually." Several studies have demonstrated that inhaled asthma medication delivered from an inhaler (MDI or DPI) is just as effective as that administered via a nebulizer, provided that a valved holding chamber is used with the MDI and the patient has mastered appropriate MDI or DPI technique. MDIs, like DPIs, are inexpensive, basically maintenance free, highly portable, and very convenient. Nebulizers are more cumbersome, require a power source, and need frequent cleaning. The same medicine that can be administered in 2 or 3 minutes by an MDI will take at least a quarter of an hour by nebulization.

There are defined circumstances when a nebulizer rather than an MDI+VHC setup or DPI might be considered. Babies and very young children (less than 5 years old) who are too young to learn inhaler technique should receive their medicine by nebulization, usually via a face mask. Most children can be taught correct MDI and DPI technique when they are of kindergarten age, particularly if there is a motivated adult in the home to supervise and encourage the child. Many of those children can also be prescribed a nebulizer to keep in reserve at home for emergency use under the guidance of a doctor in the case of a severe exacerbation. A patient of any age who cannot master correct inhaler technique will require medication administration by nebulizer. Persons who are unable to use inhalers, perhaps because of physical or neurological impairments, can usually receive their prescribed medicine via a nebulizer. Finally, some individuals with badly compromised lung function cannot inhale from an MDI deeply enough to benefit and should switch to a nebulizer. The last scenario is unusual in a person with asthma alone and is more likely with a cigarette-associated lung condition, such as advanced emphysema.

A special caution concerns nebulizer use in toddlers and young children. A child younger than 5 years must use a face mask when nebulized medication is administered.

To obtain maximal benefit from the treatment, the face mask must create a tight seal over the child's nose and mouth. Delivering nebulized medicine using what has been called the blow-by technique is totally ineffective. The blow-by method attempts to deliver medication by holding the bulb that contains the medicine under the child's nose and mouth, with the hope that it will reach the lungs. Unfortunately, it does not work! The blow-by technique does not require that you hold a mask to the child's face, so although a parent may believe they are still treating their child's asthma effectively, the fact is that only insignificant amounts of medicine reach the breathing passages.

Medications used in the treatment of asthma available in liquid form for nebulization include short-acting bronchodilators (AccuNeb, generic albuterol solution, Proventil solution, Xopenex solution), corticosteroids (Pulmicort Respules), and mast-cell stabilizers (Intal, Tilade).

69. What are corticosteroids and how do they work in asthma?

Steroids such as corticosteroids are naturally occurring chemical substances (hormones) produced by the healthy human body. The individual compounds that make up the steroid family have important roles in regulating many of the critical processes involved in our well-being. Hormones are chemical messengers produced in one organ and released into the bloodstream to exert their effects on another organ. Insulin is an example of a hormone; produced in the islet cells of the pancreas gland, it travels to the blood circulation and helps regulate glucose (sugar) uptake from food into organs such as the liver, fat tissue, and muscle. Some of the hormones our bodies make are members of the steroid family of

Hormone

A chemical messenger produced in one organ and released into the bloodstream to exert its effects on another organ.

Estrogens

A group of female hormones synthesized chiefly by the ovaries. Estrogens stimulate the development and maintenance of the female secondary sexual characteristics.

chemical compounds. The organs that produce steroid hormones are the adrenal glands, the ovaries, and the testes. During pregnancy, the placenta, an additional steroid-producing organ, develops, which produces the hormones required for the successful continuation of the pregnancy. The sex hormones estrogen and testosterone are synthesized by the ovary and testis, circulate in the bloodstream, and affect many different organs throughout the body. Similarly, the body's two adrenal glands produce adrenocortical steroids (hydrocortisone, cortisone, aldosterone, and progesterone).

Scientists have succeeded in creating (or synthesizing) steroids, including corticosteroids, in the laboratory for medical use. Corticosteroids have widespread usefulness in a diverse group of medical conditions. These steroid medicines are manufactured in different formulations to treat a variety of specific conditions. You may be surprised to learn that corticosteroid medicines are manufactured as eye drops, nasal sprays, inhalers, creams and ointments, syrups, and pills, in an intravenous form, and even as a rectal suppository. Corticosteroids are invaluable to physicians who care for persons with inflammatory eye diseases such as uveitis, skin ailments such as psoriasis and eczema, rheumatologic diseases such as rheumatoid arthritis and lupus, inflammatory bowel diseases, some kidney diseases, and, of course, several lung diseases, especially asthma.

Corticosteroids in inhaled forms are the most effective asthma controller medicines available and are recommended asthma treatment for persons of all ages, including children.

Corticosteroid medications are important because they have powerful anti-inflammatory effects; they reduce inflammation, which is the main problem in asthma and severe allergies. Corticosteroids in inhaled forms are the most effective asthma controller medicines available and are recommended asthma treatment for persons of all ages, including children. Inhaled corticosteroids are thus extensively used in asthma management and are the cornerstone of preventive therapy for all forms of persistent asthma (Table 43).

The two major physiologic reactions that characterize poorly controlled or uncontrolled asthma are bronchoconstriction and ongoing inflammation. The muscles that surround the bronchi (air passageways) go into spasm (bronchospasm), which causes the airway to narrow (bronchoconstriction). As an exacerbation progresses, several types of white blood cells including eosinophils, lymphocytes, mast cells, and neutrophils become stimulated and in turn release various chemicals called mediators. The white cell mediators cause an inflammatory reaction within the walls of the bronchial passageways. Ongoing, uncontrolled inflammation not only contributes to persistent bronchospasm, but also represents the greatest potential for causing chronic lung changes and reduced lung function in asthma. We now understand that this process can be a silent phenomenon, like high blood pressure or elevated cholesterol. A heightened inflammatory response is present to

Eosinophils

White blood cells involved in combating infection by parasites as well as playing a role in allergy and asthma.

Mediators

Chemical compounds that are either preformed or actively produced by specialized white blood cells as the result of an allergic reaction. These substances are responsible for the rapid onset of symptoms such as sneeze, runny nose, tearing eyes, cough, and wheeze, and the delayed development of inflammation.

Table 43   Inhaled Corticosteroids (ICS) in Asthma: Key Points

- ICS are manufactured as inhalers (MDI, DPI) and in solution for nebulization.
- ICS are daily-use maintenance controller medicines.
- ICS are the cornerstone of preventive therapy for all forms of persistent asthma.
- ICS use prevents symptoms of asthma from developing.
- ICS use reduces or suppresses airway inflammation.
- ICS use improves asthma-specific quality of life.
- ICS use increases lung function.
- ICS use leads to fewer lung symptoms, fewer exacerbations, and fewer severe attacks that result in hospital admission or death.

Source: Adapted from Fanta CH. Asthma. *N Engl J Med.* 2009;360:1001–1014.

some degree in every person with asthma, even in those with mild disease.

Asthma is now considered a chronic inflammatory disorder of the lungs. The response of the lungs to persistent inflammation may result in changes that never go away. The term currently used to describe this phenomenon is *airway remodeling*. Airway remodeling may contribute to declines in lung function in some persons with asthma. Lung function abnormalities seen in asthma were traditionally considered a wholly reversible phenomenon. Within the past 2 decades, our ideas about this concept have slowly evolved. There seems to be a subgroup of patients with asthma who appear to have greater degrees of inflammation in their lungs. Within that group, certain individuals' lung function never does return entirely to normal. It is unclear why exactly airway remodeling occurs. One hypothesis suggests that it results from unappreciated long-term effects of chronic asthmatic bronchial inflammation. However, the multiple factors responsible for the pathologic process called remodeling are still not completely understood. An article in the March 5, 2009, issue of *The New England Journal of Medicine* reviewed available drug therapies in asthma and noted the beneficial clinical outcomes of persons with asthma treated with inhaled corticosteroids (ICS). The authors point out that although there is no scientific evidence that ICS prevented the lung function decline observed in some persons with asthma, regular ICS use reduced or suppressed airway inflammation in asthma, increased lung function, improved asthma-specific quality of life, led to fewer asthma symptoms, fewer exacerbations, and fewer severe attacks leading to hospitalization or death. Despite overwhelming and convincing evidence of the benefits of inhaled ICS in all forms of persistent asthma, physicians are not following national guidelines

It is unclear why exactly airway remodeling occurs.

Pathologic

Abnormal finding or feature indicative of the presence of a medical condition or disease.

(such as the NAEPP's *Expert Panel Report*) for ICS prescribing in asthma!

70. My doctor wants me to take inhaled corticosteroid medication to improve my asthma control, but I am reluctant to take steroids because I heard from a friend that they are dangerous drugs. Are steroids dangerous?

No, steroids are not dangerous if taken as prescribed. Your physician has the requisite expertise to make a medically appropriate recommendation about your asthma treatment. He or she is invested in your well-being and obviously would never suggest an intervention of any sort that would harm you or not provide you with a benefit. Furthermore, every prescription medication sold in the United States has passed the FDA's rigorous approval process. Corticosteroids are no exception; like any other class of medicine, steroids are safe and effective when prescribed appropriately, and when used exactly as directed. Steroids are not inherently any more or less dangerous than other medicines. Like any other class of medicine, they do carry potential side effects, especially if used in pill form (as opposed to inhaled), long term, and in large doses. Steroid preparations have important and diverse medical uses. The development of inhaled corticosteroid medicines has revolutionized the treatment of asthma and greatly improved the quality of life of countless persons with asthma. Steroids come in formulations other than pills and inhalers. An allergic child with eczema may be treated with a steroid cream, for example. Similarly, ophthalmologists may prescribe steroid eye drops for specific conditions. Steroids are a powerful medicine in the pulmonologist's and allergist's armamentarium, and they can be truly lifesaving in

The development of inhaled corticosteroid medicines has, in particular, revolutionized the treatment of asthma and greatly improved the quality of life of countless persons with asthma.

certain medical situations, including a severe exacerbation of asthma.

Why, then, might some people erroneously think that steroids are dangerous? Some confuse anabolic steroids with corticosteroids. Anabolic steroids have been abused by some weight lifters and athletes to help them bulk up and build muscle mass, and they have a reputation for causing dangerous side effects when misused. Corticosteroids are completely different medicines than anabolic steroids and are the class of steroid medication used extensively in treatment of allergy and asthma. Another reason your friend might think of steroids as "dangerous" is that, when prescribed in oral form (pills or syrup) they have to be taken exactly as directed, in a very specific manner. If your doctor instructs you to take tapering or decreasing doses daily, for example, then you should follow the physician's directions to the letter. There are at least two important reasons for you not to stop taking the pill form of corticosteroids abruptly. The first reason is that if corticosteroids are prescribed for treatment of an exacerbation of asthma, there is a good chance that the asthma will flare anew if the steroid dosage is decreased all at once. The second reason applies in the scenario of an individual who requires steroids on a long-term basis. Our bodies all produce a form of steroids that is required for health. The right and the left adrenal glands located above each kidney are responsible for meeting the body's steroid requirements. The steroids produced by the adrenal glands are referred to as the body's "endogenous steroids." When the adrenal glands detect extra steroid medication in the bloodstream over time, they reduce their own endogenous steroid production. If the adrenal glands are exposed to a significant amount of steroid medication, they respond by completely shutting down the body's own vital manufacture

Anabolic steroids

Compounds normally produced by the healthy body that have the capacity to increase muscle mass, among other effects. Athletes have sometimes inappropriately taken anabolic steroids as supplements in order to build strength, endurance, and muscle mass.

Endogenous steroids

Steroids normally produced in health by the body's adrenal glands.

of steroids. As long as a person continues to take his or her prescribed steroid medication, the adrenals remain "lazy" and cease the production of endogenous steroids. When steroid medication is then gradually reduced, the adrenal glands have time to "wake up," and will eventually resume producing sufficient endogenous steroids for the body's needs. If, on the other hand, long-term steroid pills are stopped abruptly, the adrenal glands will not have sufficient time to recover and to restart the manufacture of endogenous steroids. The body will be left without any steroids at all, and an adrenal crisis—a true medical emergency—may ensue. The treatment of adrenal crisis requires hospital admission and includes steroid administration by the intravenous route.

Steroids are safe when taken exactly as prescribed, for bona fide medical indications. The only danger to using them occurs if they are not used correctly. If your asthma requires daily oral steroids, it is vitally important that you follow the physician's dosing recommendations. Let's say that your asthma has become less controlled. Despite the fact that you are using inhaled, long-acting β_2 agonists (LABA), along with an inhaled, high-dose corticosteroid twice a day, you are now also requiring two puffs of your quick-relief, short-acting inhaled β_2 agonist (SABA) every 4 to 6 hours for relief of breathlessness. Your peak flow values decreased yesterday and are still lower than usual today. You have been experiencing nocturnal awakenings for the past six nights because of respiratory difficulty. You feel unwell and are breathless with climbing half a flight of stairs or walking short distances. Your physician will undoubtedly prescribe a steroid burst for you. A steroid burst is a prescription for corticosteroid pills that you will take daily for a limited period of time (usually 6–21 days, depending on your asthma). You will begin with higher doses, in order to get your asthma under control, followed by gradually decreasing doses, before finally tapering off the medicine. You can expect to begin to feel an improvement in your asthma exacerbation in as little as 6 hours after the first dose of steroid pills. When used properly, steroids are truly miraculous in their effectiveness.

Prednisone and methylprednisolone (Medrol) are two different steroids in pill (or oral) form that are frequently prescribed in the treatment of asthma exacerbations and of severe allergic reactions. They are also sometimes recommended as controller therapy in very small daily doses in the treatment of severe persistent asthma. A 5-mg dose of prednisone is equivalent to a 4-mg dose of methylprednisolone (Medrol). I usually advise my patients who require steroids to start them early and get off them quickly, so they can take advantage of the beneficial qualities when treating an exacerbation and minimize potential side effects. Before inhaled formulations became available, the chronic use of oral (pill or liquid by mouth) corticosteroids was responsible for both saving many lives and causing significant side effects. Because of the availability of inhaled (and nebulized) steroids, the potential for the development of serious systemic (body-wide) side effects has decreased dramatically. Corticosteroids are pharmacologically potent; that's one reason they work so well! That said, I do not hesitate to write a prescription for an inhaled or oral steroid whenever the clinical situation is appropriate. I also carefully review the relative potential risks, anticipated benefits of the medication, and answer any questions such as the one you are posing here.

Kerrin's comment:

My son was prescribed Pulmicort Respules after being hospitalized for respiratory problems. We've been instructed to use it in the nebulizer after the albuterol (which we were told opens up the breathing passages to then allow the steroid better movement) whenever we believe his breathing is becoming compromised. It's a steroid, but it has helped keep him out of the hospital (where he would receive steroids anyway) several times, so whatever the possible side effects, they're worth it.

71. What are possible side effects of corticosteroid use?

Before answering the question, let's define what exactly side effects are. Side effects are secondary, nontherapeutic effects unrelated to the primary treatment intent of a medicine. Unlike treatment effects that occur in everyone, a side effect may or may not develop when a medicine is prescribed. Some medication side effects are unpleasant but bearable, others are limiting or harmful, and occasionally a side effect may be perceived as beneficial. Examples of each follow. A child prescribed an antibiotic to help eradicate a strep throat infection may develop loose bowel movements or some mild diarrhea while taking the antibiotic. Dietary modifications help relieve the diarrhea, which resolves soon after the antibiotic course is completed. The side effect (loose bowel movements) is not why the antibiotic was prescribed, yet the symptom can be managed effectively, and therapy can therefore continue until the child recovers from the strep infection. Sometimes, medicines cause unintended effects that are more serious, requiring discontinuance of the medication. The treatment of tuberculosis for example, usually includes a medication called isoniazid, which is known to be metabolized in the liver. Some persons (not all!) taking isoniazid can develop an inflammation of their liver, a chemical INH hepatitis. The development of INH-related hepatitis requires cessation of INH therapy at the first sign of the hepatitis. A balding

Unlike treatment effects that occur in everyone, a side effect may or may not develop when a medicine is prescribed.

middle-aged man with high blood pressure (hypertension) requiring medication for control along with his regular exercise and prudent diet, may hope that he is one of those persons who experiences new hair growth, a well-known side effect of minoxidil!

Returning to asthma therapies, the potential side effects of corticosteroids are well described in the medical literature and are related to four factors. Potential side effects are greatly minimized when corticosteroids are taken by inhalation (MDI, DPI, or nebulizer) rather than by mouth, or orally (pill or liquid) making the route of corticosteroid administration a major factor. The three other important considerations are the total daily dose taken, the total duration of steroid therapy, and an individual's particular characteristics. Keep in mind that not everyone prescribed a medicine will inevitably develop a side effect, and that fact is attributed to individual traits.

Keep in mind that not everyone prescribed a medicine will inevitably develop a side effect, and that fact is attributed to individual traits.

A person who requires a 40-mg pill of prednisone daily for 6 weeks, for example (an admittedly unusually high and prolonged dose in asthma treatment, but the kind of dose that lung specialists are used to when they treat certain non-asthma chronic lung diseases), can expect to develop different side effects than a person taking a burst of prednisone for an exacerbation of asthma. One example of a burst regimen (not the only one though!) might be 30 mg of prednisone for one day, 25 mg the next day, then 20 mg the day after, and so forth, tapering down by 5 mg each day for a total of 6 days of therapy altogether. Oral (pill form) corticosteroids may be expected to affect different people in different ways. Steroids can cause mood elevation and increased energy. Some people may experience insomnia. Steroids stimulate appetite; food tastes better. Because steroids can lead to water retention along with an increase in appetite, weight gain often occurs, particularly with longer duration of use. Steroids may cause blood pressure to rise and can cause glucose intolerance, which makes diabetes harder to control. With long-term use, steroids can lead to acne and cause the skin to bruise easily. Regular eye checkups with an ophthalmologist are important to monitor for increasing eye pressure (glaucoma) and for the development of cataracts, which may relate to longer durations of corticosteroid therapy. Some people develop a rounded facial appearance that, like some other steroid side effects, is not permanent and will disappear after the steroid medication has been tapered and discontinued. Long-term steroid treatment can lead to thinning and weakening of bone, and cause a type of osteoporosis called glucocorticoid-induced osteoporosis (GIO).

GIO is being increasingly recognized in adult respiratory patients using steroid therapies, including those treated for cigarette-related lung diseases such as emphysema. There is some uncertainty and controversy regarding what a minimum, safe, daily steroid dose is from the perspective of bone health. Clearly, steroids in pill form are of far greater concern than inhaled steroids when it comes to glucocorticoid-induced osteoporosis. Not all persons on glucocorticoids develop bone loss or GIO. Some experts quote a dose of 5 mg of prednisone by mouth daily for 3 to 6 months or more as placing a patient at risk for the development of GIO. Others quote a dose of 7.5 mg in pill form daily. One preliminary study examined bone density in adults with asthma taking inhaled steroids for 6 years and detected reduced bone density in several parts of their skeletons. GIO can be prevented or reversed with early and timely treatment. Ways to prevent and treat GIO include taking the smallest effective dose of steroids, favoring inhaled steroids for asthma treatment rather than oral steroids, adding calcium (in the range of 1200–1500 mg/day) and vitamin D (in the range of 800 to 1000 IU/day) supplements daily, performing regular weight-bearing exercise, speaking to your physician about the possible need for bone density measurement tests, and taking a class of medicines called bisphosphonates for the prevention and/or treatment of GIO, if medically appropriate. The FDA has approved risedronate (Actonel) for the prevention and treatment of GIO, and the medicine alendronate (Fosamax) for the treatment of GIO. A third medicine, zoledronic acid (Reclast) is FDA approved for the prevention and treatment of GIO in the case where daily treatment with oral glucocorticoid will be long term (more than 12 months in duration). Such long courses of treatment are not characteristic of asthma and are more likely in the treatment of rheumatologic conditions, like lupus or other autoimmune diseases.

Metered-dose inhaler (MDI)

Devices that allow the delivery of a precise and accurate dose of medicine to the lungs by inhalation. MDIs are reliable, portable, and very convenient.

Inhaled corticosteroids (ICS) have the best safety profile of all steroid preparations used to treat asthma. Inhaled corticosteroids are prescribed in one of three different forms: as an MDI, as a DPI, or as a solution to be administered through a nebulizer. Inhaled corticosteroids are cornerstone asthma medications because they are the most effective anti-inflammatory asthma treatments available. They are extremely useful maintenance controller medicines and help prevent asthma symptoms. Physicians who specialize in asthma care generally will prescribe an inhaled form of corticosteroid for maintenance or daily therapy, reserving oral (pill or liquid) steroids for treating an asthma flare or exacerbation. Possible side effects of the inhaled corticosteroids include reversible hoarseness, throat irritation, and thrush (Table 44). Thrush is a mild yeast infection that occurs in the back of the throat and looks like small white patchy blotches. Its treatment consists of an antifungal mouth rinse or occasionally a prescription for an anti-fungal pill. Using a valved holding chamber device with the MDI form of steroids, paying proper attention to careful inhalation technique, and gargling with water or a mouthwash after using the inhaler reduce the risk for developing any of the throat side effects.

All persons who inhale corticosteroids, regardless of whether the medication is administered through an MDI or DPI or by jet nebulizer, should rinse their mouth, gargle, and spit after each dose. The gargling and rinsing procedure will remove any residual steroid particles that may be trapped in the mouth or throat. If these steps are followed regularly after each dosing, the possibility of developing thrush or hoarseness decreases significantly.

You may find it practical to keep your MDI corticosteroid in the bathroom. You can then take your medication,

Table 44   Possible Side Effects of Inhaled Corticosteroid (ICS) Medication

- Greater daily doses of ICS lead to an increased risk of possible side effects as com-pared to smaller daily doses. Side effects known to be associated with sustained use of higher doses of ICS include:
  - ○ Throat effects: sore throat, cough, hoarse voice, thrush
  - ○ Skin bruising
  - ○ Eye changes (cataract formation and increased pressure in the eye)
  - ○ Slowing of growth in children
  - ○ Reduced bone mass/density
- Establishing control of asthma symptoms and maintaining control is the over-reaching principle of therapy.
- Minimizing or avoiding side effects is an important consideration in selecting an optimal asthma treatment plan.
- Physicians must be familiar with possible side effects and can advise you about what steps should be taken to reduce your chance of developing side effects and to treat them if they develop.

brush your teeth, rinse your mouth, gargle, and spit. Since you likely brush your teeth at least twice a day, you can encourage the regular use of your ICS controller medication by piggybacking onto that already established habit pattern. Note, however, that humid environments like bathrooms that become steamed up after showering are not good environments in which to store any of the DPIs. The bathroom's high humidity can cause the DPI's fine medication particles to clump together and to lose their efficacy.

One question that often comes up in treating asthma in children relates to a possible effect of inhaled steroids on a child's growth. Uncontrolled or poorly controlled asthma affects children's growth and will decrease final adult height. The most recent data show that children with asthma who are treated with inhaled corticosteroids do ultimately reach their predicted adult height, but that it is reached at a later age. In particular, current evidence indicates that the rate of a child's growth may slow during the first year of inhaled steroid use. During the second year, most children who have experienced a decreased growth rate enter a catch-up growth phase.

It is extremely important to understand that the long-term benefits associated with well-controlled asthma in virtually every case far outweigh the potential for developing harmful side effects associated with the proper use of inhaled steroids. It is a fact that poorly controlled asthma results in a long list of adverse outcomes. If you think that one of your asthma medicines, be it an inhaled corticosteroid or any another drug, is causing you to experience side effects, the next step is to review your concerns with your treating physician. It is important never to stop any prescribed medication on your own. Both the GINA and the NAEPP encourage practitioners caring for persons with asthma of any age to ask about potential medication side effects at every visit and to prescribe the smallest dose of medicine required for asthma control in order to minimize the possible risk of side effects.

PART SIX

Asthma: A Healthy Lifestyle

What are the newest approaches to the treatment of asthma?

Can acupuncture or herbal remedies help my asthma? Will alternative or complementary medicine treatments be good for my asthma?

My asthma seems to worsen each month around the time of my period. Is that possible?

Is obesity related to asthma?

What sports can persons with asthma participate in?

Is asthma mostly a psychological disease?

More . . .

72. What are the newest approaches to the treatment of asthma?

Asthma is of great interest to physicians, scientist researchers, epidemiologists, and public health experts. The National Asthma Education and Prevention Program's 440-page updated and expanded *EPR-3* published in October 2007 describes in detail the contemporary approach to the treatment of asthma. The report advises healthcare providers to treat asthma by incorporating four key components into their daily practice. The components are assessment and monitoring of asthma severity and of asthma control at every visit; education for a partnership between the person with asthma (or caregivers) and the clinician that includes self-management support; control of environmental factors and comorbid conditions that affect asthma; and the stepwise use of medications.

Currently available asthma medicines are highly effective for the majority of persons diagnosed with asthma and have an excellent safety record. As mentioned in Question 58, the inhaled route of administration is preferred, putting the medicine exactly where it is needed, while ensuring that as little active drug as possible enters other organs. It is not surprising to learn, therefore, that many recent advances relate to refining drug-delivery devices. Dry-powder inhalers were developed several decades ago and are now in widespread use worldwide. More recently, the asthma community has seen the successful development and introduction to market of the "greener" HFA (hydrofluoroalkane) propellants in MDIs, as outlined in Questions 59 and 60. As far as medications that help control and treat asthma, new approaches include the introduction of inhaled drug combinations and the development of novel drugs to treat the severest forms of persistent asthma. Combination inhalers generally contain

Hydrofluoroalkanes (HFAs)

Medically inert substances that are used as propellants in metered-dose inhalers and meet CFC-free criteria.

both an ICS (an inhaled corticosteroid) and a LABA (a long-acting β_2 agonist) bronchodilator. Examples include Advair, which contains fluticasone + salmeterol, and Symbicort, made up of budesonide + formoterol. One puff delivered from those inhalers contains two long-term daily use medicines, enhancing medication adherence and efficacy.

According to the National Heart, Lung, and Blood Institute (NHLBI) of the U.S. National Institutes of Health,

Approximately 5 to 10% of asthma patients have severe asthma that is not well controlled by long-term controller medications, such as high-dose inhaled corticosteroids, or oral prednisone. These patients may also be classified as having refractory or steroid-resistant asthma.

It emphasizes that, "new therapies are desperately needed for severe asthmatics who are poorly controlled despite . . . standard medications." One such new approach to treatment, omalizumab (Xolair), is the result of our better understanding of asthma and allergy at the molecular level. Omalizumab (Xolair) is the first clinically available drug in a new class of medicine called IgE blockers, a type of immunomodulators.

Immunoglobulin E, abbreviated IgE, is a protein that was first identified in the mid-1960s. IgE is an anti-body produced by the body in minute quantities and normally circulates in the bloodstream in very small amounts, as mentioned in Question 47. Under certain conditions, however, the body's (blood or serum) level of IgE can rise significantly. High serum IgE levels have been associated with persistent wheezing, allergy, and bronchial hyperresponsiveness. IgE plays a pivotal role in allergy, in asthma, and in the other atopic diseases, such as eczema, seasonal allergic rhinitis, peanut allergy, anaphylaxis, and hives. To better understand the central role of IgE, it is important to first review our understanding of the body's allergic response.

When a person has a medically confirmed allergy to a specific allergen, that allergy has developed over time. In order for the allergy to have emerged, several steps had to have first taken place. The initial event was allergen *exposure*, occurring earlier in their lifetime. Exposure then persisted over time, allowing the development of *sensitization* as a next step. Since the sensitized allergic individual then had a potential to react allergically, ongoing exposure to the allergen in the setting of that potential ultimately led to a clinical *allergic* response. The genesis of a specific allergy in an individual with certain innate genetic characteristics thus requires at least two preliminary steps: exposure followed by sensitization. Those two steps are necessary, but not sufficient for an allergy to emerge. Most individuals are not "allergy prone," meaning that even though they may have repeated, frequent allergen exposure, their immune system does not become sensitized, and allergic symptoms never develop.

Consider two siblings who live in a home with a cat. The older child, a boy, has no allergic symptoms. His sister however, experiences itchy eyes, runny nose, chest tightness, and wheezing when at home, and particularly when in direct contact with the family cat. The younger child was previously sensitized to the cat and now has developed allergic rhinitis and asthma triggered by her cat allergy. Her immune system has responded to the continued exposure and sensitization to cat allergen by producing antibodies directed against cat proteins. The antibodies made in the course of an allergic response are IgE antibodies, in our example, anti-cat IgE proteins. The IgE directed against cat protein is the culprit in the allergic response, causing sneeze, cough, and wheeze.

Total serum IgE level is easy to measure with a simple blood test. An elevated serum IgE level directed against a specific antigen indicates that sensitization against that antigen has occurred, but it does not automatically indicate that an allergy to that antigen is present as well. It is possible to have both an elevated total serum IgE level in the blood and no allergy symptoms at all. Before you can state that someone is allergic to something, both a positive test for the suspected allergen and a history of relevant symptoms must be present. Neither one alone is sufficient to confirm allergy. More information about testing for suspected allergy is presented in Question 46.

Before you can state that someone is allergic to something, both a positive test for the suspected allergen and a history of relevant symptoms must be present.

Scientists have been able to study and analyze the effects of IgE in humans at the cellular level. Researchers have been able to determine how the IgE interacts with effector cells in our bodies, such as macrophages, T cells, B cells, basophils, and activated mast cells, leading, in turn, to the release of substances that bring about the symptoms of an allergic response. The sophisticated research has not only advanced our understanding of how allergy and asthma develop, but has also suggested pathways for new asthma and allergy medications. In particular, a novel medication, omalizumab (Xolair), was developed specifically for patients with IgE-mediated asthma and allergy. Omalizumab binds IgE circulating in the body and so treats asthma by a unique and completely different mechanism from other existing asthma medicines. Since most of the IgE becomes bound to the omalizumab, free IgE levels are reduced. Less free IgE is available to attach to receptors found on the surface of effector cells

Effector cells

Specialized white blood cells (such as macrophages, T cells, B cells, and activated mast cells) that interact and release mediators that create the typical symptoms of an allergic response.

(mast cells and basophils), which limits the degree of release of mediators of the allergic response. Since mediator release becomes hindered, asthma and allergy symptoms are lessened. The FDA granted Xolair its approval in June of 2003, and the medicine became available in the United States by prescription a month later (Table 45). It is approved by the FDA for treatment of moderate and severe persistent asthma in adolescents and adults who meet two additional specific criteria. One is the presence of a positive skin test, or RAST blood test for a year-round allergen, such as dust mite or mold, for example. The second criterion requires that inhaled corticosteroid treatment be ineffective in adequately controlling the patient's asthmatic symptomatology.

A non-pharmacologic approach to the treatment of severe asthma, bronchial thermoplasty, is currently under investigation in Australia, Brazil, Canada, the Netherlands, the United Kingdom, and in the United States in a series

Table 45   The First in a New Class of Asthma Treatments: IgE Blockers

Omalizumab (Xolair), a medication that binds immunoglobulin E, is the prototype of a novel unique class of asthma treatment, the IgE blockers.

Omazilumab is:

- a humanized monoclonal antibody
- administered by injection, right under the skin (subcutaneous)
- taken every 2 to 4 weeks, in a doctor's office, under direct medical supervision
- dosed based on body weight and the IgE level
- FDA approved for persons 12 years of age and older
- indicated in adolescents and adults with:
  - severe persistent asthma who also have significant allergy
  - a positive skin test to a specific allergen
  - a positive RAST to a specific allergen
  - uncontrolled or poorly controlled asthma despite the use of inhaled corticosteroids
- *never* used in acute or emergency treatment of an exacerbation

of studies, collectively called the AIR trials. Bronchial thermoplasty is a minimally invasive outpatient procedure that targets airway smooth muscle with radio-frequency–generated heat. It is performed over three sessions through bronchoscopy (see Question 31 for more on bronchoscopy). Bronchial thermoplasty has been investigated in persons with severe persistent asthma that is not controlled despite high doses of inhaled corticosteroids (ICS) and long-acting β_2 agonist bronchodilators (LABA). The results of a large safety and effectiveness study (AIR-2) enrolling 297 persons at 30 sites in six countries who were followed for 1 year were published in the *American Journal of Respiratory and Critical Care Medicine* in October 2009, by the AIR2 Trial Study Group. The authors explain, "Bronchial thermoplasty (BT) is a novel intervention for asthma that delivers controlled thermal energy to the airway wall during a series of bronchoscopy procedures, resulting in a prolonged reduction in airway smooth muscle (ASM) mass." Since the amount of airway smooth muscle mass is reduced, the hypothesis is that less muscle leads to less airway narrowing from muscle constriction, which, in turn, leads to fewer exacerbations and better asthma control. The study has demonstrated that the group of persons treated with bronchial thermoplasty had "clinically meaningful improvements in severe exacerbations requiring corticosteroids, ED visits, and time lost from work/school during the post-treatment period . . . together with improvements in quality of life." The data look promising, and as of this writing, an FDA panel has recommended that the agency approve the bronchial thermoplasty device called Alair. Once approved by the FDA, it will become another treatment option for refractory, steroid-resistant asthma. Because severe persistent asthma is currently so difficult to treat, it continues to be the target of ongoing research. The work will undoubtedly not only continue to yield helpful treatments for those most severely targeted by the disease, but will ultimately provide insights into the underlying processes in asthma that will benefit anyone with asthma of any severity.

73. Can acupuncture or herbal remedies help my asthma? Will alternative or complementary medicine treatments be good for my asthma?

Scientific evidence available to date is insufficient to answer your question precisely. The term *complementary medicine* refers to treatments, practices, and products that supplement or complement traditional medical treatments. Alternative medical treatments, on the other hand, have the goal of completely replacing conventional medical therapies with alternatives. Alternative treatments essentially reject the approach to asthma we recommend. Complementary asthma therapies, on the other hand, are designed to be used alongside the asthma treatments included in this book. Some of the patients under my care for their asthma have explored yoga, swimming therapy, meditation, traditional Chinese medicine (including herbs), acupuncture, breathing exercises, and homeopathic remedies while adhering to their asthma treatment plans. In each case, we always carefully reviewed what was known about the complementary therapy, what the potential benefits and risks might be, and monitored how the complementary treatments were progressing during follow-up visits. I would never advise abandoning established asthma treatments such as bronchodilator and anti-inflammatory medicines in favor of alternative therapies. I would consider it too dangerous from a health perspective. A complementary modality, such as yoga or relaxation and breathing exercises, might instead become incorporated into your preexisting comprehensive asthma management plan. If you are interested in pursuing complementary treatments, you should begin by obtaining as much available objective, scientific evidence on the treatment as possible. You should then consult with the members of your health care team to get their advice, and keep them up to date on any decisions you make regarding your asthma care.

The National Institutes of Health (NIH) has committed to addressing "approaches to health care that are outside the realm of conventional medicine as practiced in the United States." To that end, Congress in 1998 established the National Center for Complementary and Alternative Medicine (NCCAM). The NCCAM is one of twenty-seven institutes and centers that make up the NIH. The NIH is one of eight agencies under the Public Health Service in the Department of Health and Human Services. The NCCAM states that it is "dedicated to exploring complementary and alternative healing practices in the context of rigorous science, training complementary and alternative medicine (CAM) researchers, and disseminating authoritative information to the public and professionals." In December 2008, NCCAM and the National Center for Health Statistics (part of the Centers for Disease Control and Prevention) released updated findings on Americans' use of CAM. The information is derived from data collected as part of the 2007 National Health Interview Survey (NHIS). Approximately 38% of American adults (nearly 4 in 10 on average) and 12% of children (more than 1 in 9) use some form of complementary or alternative medicine. The most commonly used therapies are nonvitamin, nonmineral, natural products, such as fish oil, glucosamine, and echinacea (the top three), followed by deep breathing techniques and meditation. Asthma is not among the top ten conditions for which Americans seek CAM. Those conditions include back pain, neck pain, joint pain, arthritis, anxiety, elevated cholesterol, chest and head colds, headaches and migraine, and insomnia. Although people of all backgrounds use CAM, its use in adults is greater among women and those with higher levels of education and higher incomes.

NCCAM is located in Bethesda, Maryland, on the NIH complex and maintains a comprehensive and informative Web site (http://www.nccam.nih.gov/) where you can obtain reliable information on alternative and complementary treatments for asthma and various other illnesses. A recent search on the NCCAM Web site for clinical trials studying complementary treatments for asthma listed 11 studies, including investigations evaluating Chinese herbal therapy, magnesium supplements, vitamin C and E, and ginkgo biloba. Recent investigations into traditional Chinese medicine, including herbal therapy, have in particular yielded very encouraging results in asthma treatment and have stimulated additional research. Objective reviews of published studies that use acupuncture to treat bronchial asthma, on the other hand, are inconclusive. The available data fails to show either clear-cut benefit or harm. The consensus among American experts is that additional high-quality research must be performed before recommendations can be made regarding the effectiveness of alternative, therapeutic approaches to asthma, hence the importance of creating clinical trials and encouraging patients to enroll in them if they are interested in CAM. The NCCAM Web site points out that "While scientific evidence exists regarding some CAM therapies, for most there are key questions that are yet to be answered through well-designed scientific studies—questions such as whether these therapies are safe and whether they work for the purposes for which they are used. NCCAM's mission is to explore CAM practices using rigorous scientific methods and build an evidence base for the safety and effectiveness of these practices."

74. My asthma seems to worsen each month around the time of my period. Is that possible?

Thirty to forty percent of women with asthma who menstruate experience exacerbation of their asthma symptoms in relation to their menstrual cycle. They consistently note increased asthma symptoms either just before or during their period. The term *premenstrual asthma* has been applied to this phenomenon. Hormonal changes, possibly related to rises in leukotriene levels, have been studied as a possible explanation for the increase in asthma symptoms. The first step in treating premenstrual asthma is to identify whether it is, in fact, present. A symptom diary together with daily peak-flow recordings can be helpful. If confirmed, premenstrual asthma can be treated with one or more of the following, depending on symptom severity and individual characteristics: stepped-up controller medicine, a trial of oral leukotriene modifiers, and in severe cases, hormone therapy or oral contraceptive medication to suppress ovulation.

75. Should I take extra vitamins or mineral supplements since I have been diagnosed with asthma?

A healthy individual who carries a diagnosis of asthma does not ordinarily require nutritional supplements on account of his or her asthma (Table 46). Asthma is a respiratory condition and does not affect your body's ability to absorb nutrients from foods. It is important to take your asthma treatment as prescribed by your physician, to exercise, and aim to keep your body weight

Table 46   Vitamin and Mineral Supplements for Asthma

- A healthy adult with asthma who eats a balanced, healthful diet will derive no additional lung benefit from taking vitamin or mineral supplements.
- Specific clinical circumstances may require consideration of vitamin and mineral supplementation. Examples include:
  - Pregnancy (may need folic acid for example, multivitamins, possibly iron)
  - Osteopenia & osteoporosis (may need extra calcium and vitamin D)
  - Food allergies that mandate elimination of a food group from the diet
  - Vegetarian diet (may require iron in some cases)
  - An exclusively breast-fed baby (will require vitamin D supplementation)
  - Persons aged 65 years and older
  - Persons with restricted calorie intake (less than 1,200 calories a day)
  - Persons with medical conditions (not asthma!) resulting in malabsorption of nutrients
- As a general rule:
  - More vitamin and mineral supplements are not necessarily better or more healthful.
  - Excess intake of fat-soluble vitamins over time can cause toxic effects.
  - Before taking any vitamin or mineral supplements, check to make sure that they will not interact adversely with your "regular" maintenance medicines or any other prescription medicine you are taking.

Your physician is a good source of medical advice regarding diet and dietary supplements; consultation with a registered dietitian (RD) may also be helpful.

Supplements should never replace good eating habits and healthful food selections.

in a healthy range by eating a well-balanced and nutritious diet. Dietary recommendations for persons without asthma obviously apply as well to individuals who also have asthma. The vitamins required for health are found in the foods we eat, with some vitamins being more abundant in the diet than others. Healthful levels of vitamin D, discussed in more detail later, may in particular be difficult to obtain from natural sources alone. A vitamin tablet you purchase in the store is synthesized in a pharmaceutical laboratory, "copied" in a sense from the vitamins extracted from food and found in nature. Supplements should never replace good eating habits and healthful food selections. Many foods in the American diet are additionally fortified with vitamins and nutrients. Vitamin D, for instance, been added to milk sold in the United States since the 1930s, in response to childhood rickets, a major childhood public health problem then. Vitamin deficiencies in our society are usually due to an illness (often of the intestinal tract or excretory system) that interferes with the body's ability to absorb the required vitamins present in food, rather than a vitamin deficiency in the diet or food itself.

A closer review of vitamins reveals that there are two categories of vitamins: fat-soluble vitamins and water-soluble vitamins. Fat-soluble vitamins include vitamins A, D, E, and K. If taken in amounts exceeding the body's immediate requirements, the extra fat-soluble vitamins are stored in the body's fatty tissues. If still more fat-soluble vitamins are ingested, vitamin toxicity can develop. Water-soluble vitamins, on the other hand, are not stored by the human body. The B vitamins and vitamin C are examples of water-soluble vitamins. If you take a tablet of vitamin C, most of it is eliminated in your urine. Your body absorbs what it requires, and the kidneys excrete the rest. Since the majority of the dose of the water-soluble vitamins Americans add to their diet in pill form ends up in their urine, many nutritionists joke that Americans have the healthiest and most expensive toilet bowl water in the world!

The U.S. National Academy of Sciences' National Research Council has established guidelines on the amount of various nutrients men and women should eat at different ages. The guidelines constitute the Recommended Dietary Allowances, or RDAs—often referred to as "Recommended Daily [sic] Allowances." In 1997, the U.S. Institute of Medicine's Food and Nutrition Board (FNB) published an updated report that modified recommendations for calcium, Vitamin D, fluoride, magnesium, and phosphorus, and eliminated the name RDA in favor of *Dietary Reference Intakes* (*DRIs*). Most healthy persons with good eating habits easily meet the DRIs.

Recommended Dietary Allowance (RDA)

Guidelines established by the United States National Academy of Sciences' National Research Council. The RDAs advise what nutrients males and females should eat at different ages. In 1997, The National Academy of Sciences' Institute of Medicine report introduced the concept of Dietary Reference Intakes (DRIs), which have supplanted the RDAs.

Adequate calcium intake is especially important in growing girls and in all teenagers. Many young people drink soda daily, often at mealtimes. The large amounts of soft drinks consumed by adolescents at the expense of milk may be one factor responsible for their increasingly inadequate calcium intake. The Institute of Medicine of the U.S. National Academy of Sciences has also added a new category, tolerable upper intake levels (ULs), to caution against excess intake of nutrients such as vitamin D that can be harmful in large amounts. You can access the latest detailed recommendations through its Web portal at http://dietary-supplements.info.nih.gov/.

What if you don't quite fit into the healthy adult with asthma eating a balanced diet category described previously? There are, of course, specific circumstances that may lead your physician to advise you to regularly supplement your diet with a multivitamin tablet or minerals. Those situations are not asthma related. For example, all pregnant women should take a folic acid supplement to help prevent neural tube defects in the developing fetus. So, it goes without saying that the recommendation for folic acid supplementation also applies to pregnant women with asthma. As this books goes to press, prior recommendations about vitamin D are undergoing intense review (Table 47). Our body obtains vitamin D from direct skin exposure to sunlight and from food in our diet. Fish oils and the flesh of fish such as salmon, tuna, and mackerel are naturally rich in vitamin D. Small amounts of vitamin D are found in beef liver, cheese, and egg yolks as well. Other food that does not naturally contain vitamin D will have it added, as in cow's milk, as mentioned previously. According to the National Institute of Health's Office of Dietary Supplements, "In the United States, foods allowed to be fortified with vitamin D include cereal flours and related products, milk and products made

Table 47   Vitamin D: New Insights

- Many persons may need to include Vitamin D–fortified foods in their diet and obtain regular sunlight exposure, while others may require additional dietary supplements to obtain adequate vitamin D levels. Groups at increased risk for developing Vitamin D deficiency include:
  - Infants who are breast-fed
  - Adults 50 years of age and older
  - Persons with limited skin exposure (home bound, northern latitudes)
  - Persons with dark skin
  - Persons with fat malabsorption (Crohn's disease, cystic fibrosis, some liver diseases)
  - Persons who are obese
  - Persons who have had gastric bypass surgery or surgery removing the upper small intestine where vitamin D becomes absorbed
- The bone disease rickets, first described in the 1600s, was known early in the 20th century to respond to two interventions, cod liver oil, and exposure to ultraviolet radiation (sunlight). The synthesis of the vitamin D molecule and better understanding of vitamin D's metabolic role are more recent developments. In the mid-1980s, researchers began to elucidate vitamin D's role in the immune system. Ongoing research has identified disease associations that merit further investigation, such as:
  - **Osteoporosis** is often associated with reduced calcium intake and insufficient levels of vitamin D contribute to reducing calcium absorption.
  - Vitamin D *could* affect **cancer** risk since laboratory, animal, and epidemiological studies *suggest* (but do not prove) that it may protect against the development of certain types of colon, and perhaps breast and prostate cancers.
  - Vitamin D may play a role in the prevention and treatment of some forms of **diabetes** & **glucose** intolerance.
  - Vitamin D may play a role in the prevention of certain forms of **hypertension**.
  - Vitamin D deficiency *may* be associated with an increased incidence of **asthma** symptoms in children.
  - Research is underway to confirm if higher maternal intakes of vitamin D during pregnancy are associated with decreased risks for recurrent wheeze in young children.
- Measurement of vitamin D is performed through a blood test and a deficiency is simple to detect.

Source: Adapted from the NIH's Office of Dietary Supplements factsheet on Vitamin D, accessed at http://ods.od.nih.gov/factsheets/vitamind.asp

from milk, and calcium-fortified fruit juices and drinks. Maximum levels of added vitamin D are specified by law." Identification of groups of people at risk for vitamin D deficiency, recognition of wide-ranging adverse health outcomes from vitamin D deficiency, and determination of appropriate and safe supplementation strategies are the focus of active research. Recent developments are summarized in Table 47.

In 2008, the American Academy of Pediatrics (AAP) issued recommended intakes for vitamin D that exceed those of the Food and Nutrition Board. "Prevention of Rickets and Vitamin D Deficiency in Infants, Children, and Adolescents," published in *Pediatrics*, the journal of the American Academy of Pediatrics, advised vitamin D supplementation for all breast-fed infants and for youngsters and teenagers who do not obtain 400 I.U. daily of vitamin D through their diet. The Food and Nutrition Board then established an expert committee in 2008 to review the DRIs for vitamin D and calcium to determine safe upper limits for both and revise, if necessary, the DRIs last published in 1997. The updated Food and Nutrition Board report is expected in May 2010.

Of particular importance for the reader is the person with severe food allergy who requires the elimination of an entire food group. A child with a peanut allergy does not need to compensate for the lack of peanuts in his diet, for example, but another child unable to drink milk or eat cheese certainly should be placed on calcium supplements to ensure an adequate intake of calcium. Finally, if your calorie intake is reduced or limited (by dieting or loss of appetite) below 1200 calories (as a general cut off), you probably should take a multivitamin and mineral supplement on a regular basis. Be sure to check with your doctor if you think you may require vitamin or mineral supplements.

76. Is obesity related to asthma?

A relationship between obesity and asthma continues to stimulate medical interest (Table 48). Physicians as well as the public have long postulated a link between obesity

Obesity

The condition of being significantly overweight. A person is obese if he or she weighs more than 30% above his or her ideal body weight for his or her given age, height, and gender. Another definition of obesity involves computation of the BMI. An overweight adult has a BMI of between 25 and 30, while an obese adult has a BMI of 30 or greater.

Table 48   Asthma and Obesity

- Both asthma and obesity affect millions of Americans.
- Increasing rates of obesity have risen in parallel with increasing asthma rates.
- Asthma and obesity often co-exist in an individual.
- Epidemiologic studies have confirmed an association between asthma and obesity.
- Obesity is associated with asthma persistence and severity in children and in adults.
- Obesity *may* be a risk factor for the development of asthma, especially in young women, but the exact mechanism is unclear, despite ongoing research.
- Obese adults with asthma who lose weight have
  - improvements in lung function tests (FEV_1)
  - reduced exacerbations
  - less need for oral corticosteroids
  - improvement in quality of life
- Overweight and obese persons with asthma should understand that weight loss will improve their overall health and may improve asthma control.

and asthma. The prevalence of both obesity and asthma are rising in parallel in Western societies. Several human population studies have demonstrated an association between being overweight and the likelihood of carrying an asthma diagnosis. Yet, the precise relationship between the two conditions remains controversial.

Does asthma cause obesity? Does obesity cause asthma? Or, is there a common underlying factor that causes both asthma and obesity? The scientific pulmonary community has started to tackle the questions.

One traditional theory maintains that asthma, particularly less than optimally managed asthma, leads to a more sedentary lifestyle. According to the theory, some persons with asthma do not exercise, either because of a mistaken belief that exercise is bad for asthma or because their asthma is not well controlled and flares with exercise. Because of lack of exercise, they become more out of shape, more sedentary, gain more weight, and ultimately may become obese.

An alternative theory suggests that obesity is the primary event. Fat tissue is not inert but is metabolically active. The theory holds that the obese state leads to the generation of inflammatory mediators that, in turn, cause changes in the lungs and airways, and ultimately asthma. Both theories have their merits, but neither one satisfactorily explains why asthma does not affect males and females equally. A third, more contemporary approach, with intriguing supportive data in laboratory animals, attempts to sort out the influence of chromosomal changes and hormonal factors that might confer predispositions to both asthma and overweight status. In 1994, a protein molecule called leptin was identified in humans. Leptin is primarily produced by fatty tissues. Leptin and a second protein called ghrelin are both suspected of playing important roles in the regulation of food intake, energy balance, and ultimately of weight. Of interest to lung researchers, lung and airway cells appear to carry receptors for leptin on their surfaces, and leptin furthermore stimulates the proliferation of the lung and airway cells, acting as a kind of stimulatory lung growth factor. Some preliminary studies in humans have documented elevated blood leptin levels in certain types of marked obesity, but research that is more recent has failed to confirm a link with the development of asthma.

Leptin

A human protein identified in 1994 and named after leptos, the Greek word for thin. Leptin seems to play a role in the regulation of food intake, energy balance, and ultimately of weight.

A key to better understanding the obesity–asthma link may come from the study of girls and boys in puberty and adolescence. More than 1000 babies born between May 1980 and January 1984 were entered at birth in the ambitious and ongoing Tucson Children's Respiratory Study. Nearly 1300 youngsters enrolled in the study and have been followed and reassessed at regular intervals for over 20 years by Dr. Fernando Martinez and his team.

The study was designed to study respiratory health and illness over time, in a prospective fashion. In particular, the development of asthma was carefully evaluated. In 2001, Dr. Martinez and his coworkers reported that girls who became overweight or obese between the ages of 6 and 11 years of age had an increased risk for developing new asthma symptoms during early adolescence. They found that girls—but not boys—who became overweight between 6 and 11 years of age were 5–7 times more likely to develop new asthma symptoms at ages 11 and 13, compared to girls who did not become overweight or obese at ages 6 and 11 years. Boys who became significantly overweight between 6 and 11 years of age did not exhibit an increased risk for the development of asthma or asthma-like symptoms. The strongest association between overweight status and asthma risk was seen in females who underwent puberty before the age of 11 years. Being overweight is associated with earlier onset of puberty. Could there be a common factor that leads to overweight status in girls, followed by early puberty and then the development of asthma? The findings are especially interesting because it has long been observed that new cases of asthma in females are especially common in the adolescent years. Further, the male: female ratio (2:1) of asthma seen in young, school-age children changes over to a female preponderance by adulthood. A role for female hormones has long been suspected, and the data from the Tucson Children's Respiratory Study supports this theory and suggests avenues for further research.

Puberty

The time during which sexual maturation occurs. Also refers to the time when reproductive organs develop to allow reproduction.

Apart from the links between obesity and asthma risk, being overweight is medically undesirable. Even my patients with very well-controlled asthma symptoms report that their breathing is much "easier" when they maintain a comfortable weight. They feel more limber, less achy, and describe greater endurance. It makes sense that if you carry excess weight on your frame, it literally feels as if you are transporting additional pounds as you walk around. Studies in adults have demonstrated that weight loss in overweight persons with asthma improves lung function, reduces exacerbations, decreases the need for oral corticosteroids (bursts), and leads to enhancements in quality of life measures. Everybody with asthma must know their weight, their height, and understand what a healthy weight is for them. The CDC's Web site points out that "Overweight and obesity are both labels for ranges of weight that are greater than what is generally considered healthy for a given height. The terms also identify ranges of weight that have been shown to increase the likelihood of certain diseases and other health problems."

Body mass index (BMI)

A mathematical formula based on height and weight. BMI is a tool used in population studies of obesity because of its ease of measurement. The BMI in most individuals correlates to measures of body fat.

How can you tell whether you are overweight or obese? One way is to determine your body mass index (BMI) once you know your height and weight. An adult with a BMI of 25 to 29.9 falls into an overweight category and one whose BMI is equal to or greater than 30 is considered obese. Healthy BMI values range from 18.5 to 24.9, and persons with BMIs less than 18.5 are underweight. BMI is a measure that also applies to children. The mathematical formula for calculating BMI is your weight (in kilograms) divided by the square of your height (in centimeters). If you know your height in inches and your weight in pounds, simply divide your weight (in pounds) by the square of your height (in inches) and multiply that result by 703. If you prefer not to do the math, there are many Web sites that will do it for you! Simply go to your preferred search engine, and type a phrase such as "ideal body weight calculator," or "BMI computation" to find a BMI calculator. Enter the data it requests, such as your weight (in pounds or kilograms), height (in inches or centimeters), and age, and then sit back as it calculates your BMI. The definitions of overweight and obesity for children and teenagers are different from the adult definitions. Age-and sex-specific pediatric BMI charts are used to determine if a child is overweight or obese. You must obtain a table of predicted BMI for children to compare your child's BMI to the standard, or you may use the CDC's calculator at http://apps.nccd.cdc.gov/dnpabmi/Calculator.aspx. A child with a BMI greater or equal to the 85th percentile and less than the 95th percentile is overweight. One whose BMI is equal to or greater than the 95th percentile for his or her age, height, and weight is considered obese. A child would be considered severely obese if his or her BMI was greater or equal to the 95th percentile.

You can also get a general idea of how your weight compares to an ideal by estimating how far off from predicted values your weight is. The formula for calculating an adult's ideal body weight requires knowledge of your height. Females are allowed 100 pounds for the first 5 feet of height, and 5 more pounds for each additional inch above 5 feet. A few additional pounds are added or subtracted for persons with large or small frames. Therefore, a 5′3″ woman should ideally weigh about 115 pounds, which corresponds to a BMI of between 20 and 21, well within a healthy range. The formula for men is similar; a man is allowed 106 pounds for the first 5 feet of height, and 6 additional pounds are added for every additional inch over 5 feet. A 6-foot tall man of average build would thus be expected to weigh 178 pounds, yielding a BMI of 25, within the desirable range. As for women, there is a correction for individuals with small and large frames.

77. Is caffeine good for people with asthma?

Caffeine is a naturally occurring compound. The German analytical chemist Friedrich Ferdinand Runge

Caffeine

A naturally occurring compound found in coffee and tea and added to other beverages such as soda or energy drinks. It is also added to some medications, such as those used for treatment of pain or headache.

(1795–1867) discovered caffeine in 1819, apparently at the urging of Gœthe, who had encouraged Runge to study and analyze coffee. We now know that caffeine is naturally present in foods such as coffee beans, tea leaves, cacao beans (used to make chocolate), kola nuts, guarana, and maté. Caffeine is also frequently added to beverage products, such as carbonated soft drinks and drinks marketed as energy drinks. It is also available in pill form, either alone (NoDoz, Vivarin), or as an additive, to aspirin for example, as in Anacin and Excedrin.

Research studies of the effect of caffeine in humans confirm that caffeine is a bronchodilator. It improves pulmonary function, and although it is a weak bronchodilator, it clearly has beneficial effects on direct measurements of lung function, such as the vital capacity, the FEV_1, and expiratory flows (discussed in Question 28). Studies of the human metabolism of caffeine reveal that ingested caffeine is metabolized by the body and transformed into three separate compounds. Caffeine metabolites are paraxanthine, theobromine, and theophylline. Theophylline is a well-known bronchodilator, used in pill form for decades in the treatment of several lung ailments, including asthma, chronic obstructive bronchitis, and emphysema. The effects of orally administered caffeine are maximal at about 2 hours after ingestion and wear off after approximately 6 hours. Incidentally, if you are undergoing pulmonary function testing as part of an evaluation of possible asthma, you should avoid caffeine for at least 4 hours prior to lung testing. So, to get back to the question about caffeine being good for people with asthma—if you enjoy caffeinated beverages, know that the caffeine they contain will, if taken in high enough doses, provide bronchodilatation and possibly modestly improve your lung function. Sounds good to me!

Bronchodilatation

A widening or opening up of the lung air passages; the reverse of bronchoconstriction. Bronchodilator medicines improve breathing and relieve asthma symptoms by opening and restoring the caliber of abnormally narrowed (constricted) bronchi.

78. What sports can persons with asthma participate in? Is it better to use my inhaled asthma medication before or after I work out? What sports are especially beneficial for asthma?

People with asthma can participate in many sports—as long as their asthma is well controlled! Exercise is a potential symptom trigger for the majority of people with asthma, be they adults or children, weekend warriors or elite athletes. Studies estimate that nearly 80% of persons with a diagnosis of asthma develop one or more symptoms of cough, breathlessness, or wheezing from exercising. Those individuals have, by definition, incompletely treated asthma. If your asthma interferes with your ability to exercise, then your asthma requires better control. Asthma specialists will make a distinction between a person with asthma in whom exercise is one of several triggers, and a person who only experiences asthma symptoms in the setting of exercise. The latter individual probably carries a diagnosis of exercise-induced bronchospasm, or EIB (reviewed in Question 36). Remember that well-controlled asthma is compatible with a full and active lifestyle (discussed in Question 42). If you do experience exercise-related symptom flares of asthma, your asthma treatment needs improvement and fine tuning. An improved treatment regimen does not automatically mean that you require additional medicine. You may require a change as simple as taking your medicine earlier in the day, or before you exercise. Just as importantly, an improved treatment regimen does not mean that you should no longer exercise or participate in sports that you enjoy. An interesting fact about asthma and exercise is that exercise itself is a bronchodilator! With exercise, the lungs' passages actually dilate and open up more. Exercise is good for your lungs! You have

If your asthma interferes with your ability to exercise, then your asthma requires better control.

With exercise, the lungs' passages actually dilate and open up more. Exercise is good for your lungs!

a responsibility to report any exercise-related symptoms to your physician or asthma specialist. Your treating doctor has a responsibility, in turn, to address the emergence of exercise-related symptoms and advise you on appropriate measures and treatment.

Successful treatment of asthma always includes a prescription for aerobic exercise. A balanced exercise program, tailored to a person's specific interests and abilities, is ideal and inherent to good health. Exercise can be separated into aerobic, flexibility, and anaerobic activities. The first achieves cardiopulmonary fitness, the second targets the range of muscle and joint motion, and the third focuses on muscle buildup and strength. Pedaling a bicycle is an example of aerobic exercise. As you pedal faster, your heart and lungs work in tandem to provide oxygen to exercising muscles while excreting acids from the accumulating effort. Yoga is an example of a flexibility exercise. Weightlifting is an anaerobic exercise. A good exercise regimen can incorporate a balance of all three types of exercise, with particular emphasis on aerobic activities.

Studies have identified factors that tend to trigger asthma symptoms during exercise. A leading hypothesis implicates the rapid inhalation of dry, cold air as the major contributor to exercise-induced asthma. Mouth breathing, in particular, bypasses the nasal passages, which serve to warm and moisten inhaled air before it enters the lungs. Another contributor to exercise symptoms is obvious, but all too common: poor adherence to treatment. In other words, if you are not taking your prescribed asthma medicine and you are experiencing flares in your asthma symptoms, then going outdoors to snowshoe through the woods on your winter vacation, for example, will undoubtedly provoke additional symptoms! Make sure that your asthma is under control before exercising. Apart from taking your medicines, you may find it useful to measure your peak flow and use the PEF value to make an objective decision about participation in sports that day.

The third factor in exercise-induced asthma relates to the type of exercise itself. Some types of exercise are especially advisable in the setting of asthma, while others are viewed as more likely to trigger asthma. In the latter category, distance running or cross-country skiing, for example, can cause symptoms of cough, breathlessness, or wheezing. Distance running, cycling, and Nordic skiing involve very good aerobic conditioning, but the activity is steady, without breaks or interruption, and includes exposure to the outdoors, with extremes of temperature, aeroallergens, and sometimes atmospheric pollutants as well. Athletic activity that incorporates breaks in the intensity of exertion is less likely to cause asthma symptoms by, in a very real sense, allowing time for you to catch your breath. Examples include competitive sports such as tennis, soccer, field hockey, basketball, baseball, and lacrosse. I encourage exercise and sports for all of my patients. The fact that distance activities have been shown in research studies to be more likely to provoke exercise-induced asthma symptoms in no way leads me to discourage my patients with asthma from cycling, running in a marathon, or cross-country skiing, if they so desire. My patients tell me what athletics they want to participate in. My job is to help control their asthma and allow them full and satisfying participation in their chosen exercise routine.

Parents sometimes want to know what sport to encourage for their child with asthma. Swimming is an excellent form of exercise for persons of any age with asthma. The warm and humid air in indoor swimming is especially gentle for asthmatic lungs and unlikely to trigger symptoms. Swimming is also outstanding aerobic exercise. It develops muscle groups symmetrically, and helps develop a healthy awareness of breathing while increasing a person's overall fitness and well-being. Since swimming is not a contact sport, musculoskeletal injuries are rare. Note, too, that swimming is a form of exercise that you never grow out of. It is truly a forever sport! Be aware that swimming in a cold atmosphere, in water that is too cold, or in a heavily chlorinated pool can trigger asthma. Ozone treatment and disinfection of swimming pools has been commonly practiced in Europe for over 50 years, and is slowly being introduced and accepted in the United States. Swimming pools disinfected primarily with ozone have enhanced water clarity, along with greatly reduced chemical odors. The pool water is purer and far less irritating to skin, eyes, and lungs. If you live in an area with a choice of pools, you may want to research whether any of the pools are primarily disinfected with ozone. The first commercial indoor pool in the state of New York to be primarily disinfected by ozone for example, is located at the 92nd Street Y in Manhattan.

To successfully incorporate exercise and sports in your asthma treatment, keep your asthma well controlled, consult with your physician regarding any special exercise or sport-specific required measures, and build up to your desired level of activity gradually and steadily. Additional, more specific recommendations focus on preventive measures before each exercise session. Several inhaled asthma medications are especially useful when administered preventively, shortly before exercise. The medicines include the inhaled, short-acting β_2 agonists, as well as inhaled cromolyn and nedocromil. Depending on the degree of your asthma and what your maintenance treatment is, your asthma might greatly benefit from a dose of inhaled medicine before exercise. It is far better, and medically more desirable, to take an inhaled medicine for your asthma before exercise than it is to attempt exercise and develop any combination of breathlessness, cough, chest tightness, uncomfortable breathing, or wheezing. If symptoms occur, chances are that you will not achieve a satisfying workout and may even have to stop prematurely. You will then be in the position to play catch-up in your attempt to treat the emerging symptoms. If your doctor instructs you to administer two puffs of an inhaler in the setting of exercise, take the inhalations before your workout to protect your lungs and to prevent exercise-induced symptoms.

Let's say that you have intermittent asthma and are treated with as-needed, inhaled, short-acting β_2 agonist medication. Your asthma symptoms have been extremely well controlled. You now notice that you are developing asthma symptoms on the days that you participate in an aerobic dance class. You are then instructed to inhale two puffs of the inhaled medicine 30 minutes before your dance class to protect your lungs. The results are striking. Not only does your asthma become controlled, but now you are able to keep up with the instructor and her demanding moves.

Another clinical scenario takes advantage of the fact that the leukotriene modifier class of asthma treatment is also very helpful in the treatment of exercise-induced bronchospasm (EIB). A fit, young man recently consulted me because of cough. On his first office visit, he explained that he had set his sights on running a marathon. He was very knowledgeable about running techniques and had embarked on a well-planned training regimen after work and on weekends. As he continued to train, he developed an episodic cough. It turned out that my future

Leukotriene

An inflammatory molecule.

marathoner had two diagnoses: seasonal allergic rhinitis (hay fever) and exercise-induced bronchospasm (EIB). He was determined to achieve his goal of becoming a distance runner and competing in a few marathon races. I was determined to treat his symptoms and control the EIB. I am happy to report that we both achieved our goals! I treated him with a once-daily tablet of montelukast (Singulair), one of the leukotriene modifier medicines. On cold winter days, when he insisted on running outdoors despite the inauspicious weather, he premedicated with two puffs of an inhaled, short-acting β_2 agonist before his warm-up. He was happy and not coughing; I was happy with his lung function, and he was able to compete in and finish both the New York City and Boston marathons.

In addition to inhaling any preventive and protective asthma medicine, always perform a warm-up before exercising and a cool-down afterwards. The warm-up activity takes advantage of the fact that exercise is a bronchodilator. When you warm up, your goal is to perform enough activity to allow the bronchial tubes to open up a bit more. Depending on your sport, you should perform about 10 minutes of light exertion, enough to break a sweat. You could, for instance, do repeated, brief (10–30 second) sprints. Stop exercising immediately after you complete your warm-up, and then wait for at least 30 minutes before getting down to your "real" exercise. Avoid cold air as much as possible. Cover your nose and mouth during outdoor sports in cool air to help warm the air you inhale. Some people like to wear a scarf or pull a neck gaiter over their mouth to keep warm. If you are a runner, switch to an indoor treadmill in a heated gym on very cold days. Similarly, if you live in an area with significant air pollution at certain times of the year, consider moving your workout indoors on those days. Most daily newspapers publish measures of air quality on the weather page. If your area is subject to a day or more of atmospheric ozone alerts during hot, muggy summer days, pay attention, protect your lungs and move the exercise indoors. Similar advice applies if you have allergic asthma triggers such as tree or grass pollens. If you are planning to exercise outdoors, and the atmosphere has high air concentration of specific allergens that you know trigger your asthma, use your common sense. Try to prevent an allergic flare and consider moving the activity to an indoor, air-conditioned venue.

In conclusion, well-controlled asthma is no barrier to fitness and sport. If you require inhaled medicine, make certain you take it before exercise, even if your PEF is normal and you feel fine. Remember to warm up and cool down. View your physician as your ally, and report any concerns you may have about exercising with asthma.

Gemma's comment:

I walk several mornings a week with a friend my own age. Although this exercise is not particularly strenuous, I always take my inhaled medication before I leave home, because we walk in the morning, when the streets are likely to be dusty, sweepers and garbage trucks are out, and, in the spring and fall, pollen and leaf particles are in the air. I'm also a regular participant in aerobic class at a neighborhood gym. I find that a routine that includes warm-up stretches, about half an hour of more rapid movement, some weight lifting and some mat work is good for overall toning, as well as mood and relaxation. Although the indoor air of the gym is rather stuffy, I don't need inhaled medication when I work out there. In fact, if I'm getting over a cold and feel some tightness in the chest, I find crunches especially helpful. The curled-up position gives just enough compression to loosen some obstruction in the lungs and make breathing easier.

My daughter recommends pranayama yoga (breathing exercises) to ease asthma symptoms. We both recognize that swimming and other aquatic routines protect joints and may offer a good aerobic workout, but we also agree that we have never used a pool that does not, sooner or later, cause itchy skin, reddened eyes, and troubled breathing.

79. How should I pack my asthma medicine in anticipation of air travel?

Always, always, always place your medicine in your carry-on bag when you travel by air.

Always, always, always place your medicine in your carry-on bag when you travel by air. One obvious reason is that you may need to use your inhaled asthma medicine during the flight, or at the airport, and you will want to have it handy. You should not pack medicine in your checked luggage. Checked suitcases are stored in the hold of the aircraft. The hold is not always heated and pressurized to the same extent that the passenger cabin is. Most medicine needs to be kept at room temperature. Also, checked suitcases are frequently waylaid or lost, unlike a bag you keep in your possession. Imagine what a vacation would be like if your medicine arrived 3 days after you did!

Before you travel, make sure that you have enough of your prescription asthma and allergy medicines to last for the duration of your trip. You should bring all your usual daily use maintenance asthma drugs with you, as well as any quick-relief inhalers that you use on an as-needed basis. You should also travel with epinephrine auto-injectors (Epi-Pen, Twinject) if you have experienced anaphylaxis from severe allergy. Auto-injectors are permitted in carry-on luggage, but they must be in the original packaging, with the pharmacy's dispensing label still affixed. As of this writing, the Transportation Security Administration (TSA) requests that you declare the epinephrine by notifying the security screeners at the security

Epinephrine

A naturally occurring hormone produced by the human adrenal glands. A synthetic form (adrenaline) is used to treat severe allergic reactions (anaphylaxis) and life-threatening asthma.

checkpoint that you are carrying auto-injectors for your medical condition. You are not required to travel with a letter from your physician confirming the medical necessity of traveling with auto-injectors, but many physicians will gladly write you such a letter if you ask them to. You can obtain the latest information on traveling by air with medicines at the TSA Web site (www.tsa.gov), and in particular at http://www.tsa.gov/travelers/airtravel/specialneeds/. Nebulizers are permitted in carry-on bags; any batteries must be disconnected, and the machine cannot be used in flight. The patient's name on any prescription's label must match the passenger's identification papers. Also, if your travels take you outside of the United States, it is a good idea to check in with your physician ahead of time to see if there are any additional medicines you should bring along, such as corticosteroids, antibiotics, or epinephrine. Even though communication by phone anywhere in the world is now easily achieved, obtaining a prescription medication on a moment's notice in a country far away from your doctor can become very complicated.

80. I am traveling to the Caribbean on vacation and plan to go scuba diving, but my husband says it's not safe since I have asthma. What guidance can you give us?

In the past, asthma of any type and of any severity was viewed as an absolute contraindication to scuba diving. Scuba diving requires inhalation of dry, compressed air through a mouthpiece, which many people find uncomfortable. The biggest concern for a diver with asthma is of course, having an exacerbation under water. Studies suggest that asthma increases a diver's risk of developing complications, such as arterial gas embolism, barotrauma, and decompression sickness. Asthma places an individual at increased risk of diving complications because of the

Air trapping

A potentially reversible phenomenon that develops in the lungs of patients with poorly controlled or uncontrolled asthma. Air trapping can be detected on chest CT scans but is best assessed by pulmonary function test measurements.

potential for air trapping, bronchospasm, and mucous plugging in asthmatic airways. Persons with asthma were thus issued a total prohibition and always advised that scuba diving was off limits, although snorkeling on the surface was acceptable. Today, with careful medical screening and medical preparation, some individuals with well-controlled, stable asthma who have normal spirometry and who understand the increased risks can go scuba diving, after a detailed medical evaluation and clearance by a physician familiar with diving and asthma. Studies performed by physicians with a specialty in diving medicine in the United States and abroad have yielded specific recommendations and guidelines. For example, people with exercise-induced bronchospasm (EIB) or cold-induced bronchospasm should not dive. Similarly, any person with asthma who requires inhalation of an inhaled β_2 agonist, quick-relief inhaler should be prohibited from diving until at least 48 hours have elapsed without a need for a dose of the bronchodilator medication.

I would need to know more about your asthma, your overall level of health and fitness, as well as your swimming and diving skills. Common sense suggests that if you have never had scuba diving instruction, vacation is not a good time to start diving with asthma. Similarly, if your asthma is not controlled on vacation, you should not dive. An alternative approach would be to first consult with your physician and undergo any appropriate testing and evaluation. Then, with your physician's approval, you could enroll in scuba classes taught by certified professionals. The Professional Association of Diving Instructors (PADI) maintains a Web site, http://www.padi.com/scuba/, where you can locate classes in your hometown. You can also learn more about diving with asthma and its risks at DAN, the Divers Alert Network, at http://www.diversalertnetwork.org. Physicians (myself included!) take the approach that safety always comes first. At the risk of appearing to side with your spouse, if pressed for an answer, I would advise you not to scuba dive on your Caribbean trip and enjoy another sport instead.

81. What is influenza? Why should I get a flu shot (influenza vaccination)? Will the flu shot make me ill?

Influenza is a serious respiratory disease caused by the influenza virus (Table 49). Influenza viruses are classified as types A, B, or C. Influenza A, the most common, is the type of influenza that causes most serious epidemics. Influenza viruses of B type have also been responsible for epidemics of seasonal influenza illness, but tend to lead to milder illness than the A viruses. Influenza produces widespread, sporadic respiratory illness each year during fall and winter in the Northern Hemisphere. It has also been known to occur in epidemic or pandemic forms, most recently in 2009. That year, a novel influenza A virus–the 2009 H1N1–emerged in the Western Hemisphere. On June 11, 2009, Dr. Margaret Chan, director-general of the World Health Organization (WHO), announced that the 2009 H1N1 virus had become a worldwide pandemic. At the time, more than 70 countries had reported cases of H1N1 infection with ongoing outbreaks of the newly identified and novel H1N1 in multiple parts of the world. WHO accordingly raised the worldwide pandemic alert to Phase 6, its highest. H1N1 became a top priority for physicians and scientists, especially public health experts, epidemiologists, virologists, and vaccine experts. It was quickly apparent that some groups were at increased risk of complications, including death, from H1N1 infection. Those groups included children, adolescents, pregnant women, persons with asthma

Asthma: A Healthy Lifestyle

Virus

A type of infectious agent. Viruses contain a single strand of either DNA or RNA, surrounded by a protein coat.

Influenza

The influenza virus and the infectious illness caused by that virus. Influenza begins abruptly and is characterized by high fever, chills, aches, and exhaustion.

Epidemic

An outbreak of a disease that spreads abnormally quickly and extensively.

Pandemic

An epidemic that has spread extensively, affecting most countries and regions of the globe.

Vaccine

A specialized preparation designed to stimulate the body's immune system to make protective antibodies directed against a specific infectious agent. Some vaccines are injected into muscle or skin; others are inhaled or swallowed.

Table 49   Influenza Quick Facts

- Any person with asthma who becomes ill from influenza has a greater chance of developing serious health complications from influenza (as compared to someone without asthma).
- The CDC estimates that 5% to 20% of the American population becomes ill with seasonal influenza each year, 200,000 persons (including 20,000 children) are hospitalized for treatment of complications, and about 36,000 persons die from seasonal influenza.
- The best way to prevent influenza infection ("the Flu") is immunization—every year in the fall.
- Every person with asthma is a candidate for yearly influenza vaccination (unless they have an absolute medical contraindication, such as for example, an allergy to egg).
- People with asthma should receive the injected influenza vaccine ("a shot") that contains a killed form of the virus. The nasal (spray) vaccine is not appropriate for persons with asthma.
- There are two vaccines approved for use in the United States. The influenza vaccine given by injection is made from a killed form of the virus and therefore cannot transmit or "cause" influenza.
- If you have asthma and symptoms of influenza, call your doctor right away to review your symptoms and obtain guidance regarding both any required treatment and measures to keep your asthma controlled.
- Although anti-viral medication may be prescribed to treat an influenza infection, prevention of infection remains the best strategy in combating flu.
- Anti-viral medication can be helpful if taken within 48 hours of onset of influenza symptoms.
- Antibiotics are not effective against the influenza virus.
- *Never* give a child or teenager with influenza or flu symptoms aspirin (acetylsalicylic) acid.
- People with influenza are infectious and can spread the infection to others beginning one day before they develop symptoms and for at least five days after becoming sick.
- If you become ill with influenza, protect those around you! Stay home from work or school, keep away from others as much as possible, avoid touching your eyes, nose, and mouth, wash your hands often with soap and water, cough and sneeze into a disposable tissue and throw it into the trash after use!

and with other underlying health conditions, such as obesity, diabetes, and immune deficiency.

Influenza disease is completely different from the common cold. Influenza is a specific respiratory illness, caused by one of the influenza viruses. Many people wrongly say that they "have the flu" to indicate that they are under the weather or ill in a general sort of way. The symptoms of seasonal influenza include the sudden, abrupt onset of chills and high fever in the range of 102°F to 103°F. Severe, generalized aches and pains, often most intense in the back and the legs, accompany the fever. Exhaustion is common, as is headache and loss of appetite. Pain felt behind the eyeballs is often reported. Respiratory symptoms are initially mild; a scratchy or sore throat can accompany a slight dry cough. The lung symptoms develop later and come to dominate the picture with persistent and productive cough as an unmistakable feature. Fever can last up to 5 days in uncomplicated cases. After other symptoms subside, weakness and fatigue may linger for several weeks.

Unfortunately, not all persons who become ill with influenza have an uncomplicated course as just described. Severe, fulminant, or fatal pneumonia can complicate influenza. Seasonal influenza is responsible for more than 36,000 deaths and 200,000 hospitalizations each year in the United States alone. Many of the deaths and hospitalizations occur among persons with underlying health conditions that place them at increased risk for complications. Increasing age (age 50 years or older), as well as very young age (age 2 years or younger) also place individuals at increased risk of influenza complications. Pregnancy is a common and often underestimated risk for complications from influenza infection. Asthma is also considered a potential risk. Influenza can now be diagnosed in a few minutes in a doctor's office. If you have symptoms of influenza, your doctor may advise you to have a nasal wash performed to be tested for the influenza virus. Your physician will let you know if you are a candidate for immediate treatment with an antiviral medicine. The available medications include oseltamivir (Tamiflu), which is FDA approved for treatment of influenza for

Fulminant

Occurring suddenly, with great intensity and severity.

those aged 1 year and older, and zanamivir (Relenza), which is approved for older children and adults. Since zanamivir is administered by inhalation, it is generally not recommended for persons with asthma, as it may cause wheezing. Both medicines shorten the time period during which you can transmit influenza to others and help to reduce the severity and duration of your illness, provided they are taken very early in the course of influenza. Oseltamivir, for example, is effective only if started within 48 hours of the onset of influenza symptoms. Taking either medicine later in the course of an established influenza infection does not provide benefit. Oseltamivir is also approved for the prevention (prophylaxis) of influenza in exposed and at-risk adults, as well as adolescents aged 13 years and older. Neither oseltamivir nor zanamivir is considered a substitute for influenza vaccination.

The single best way to prevent influenza is vaccination.

The single best way to prevent influenza is vaccination (Table 50). Vaccination against influenza virus causes the body's immune system to manufacture protective antibodies. The antibodies produced in response to successful vaccination will help fight off influenza when and if a person becomes exposed to the virus. Detailed studies of the structure of the influenza virus reveal that the virus wraps itself in a protective envelope or coat. Different strains of influenza virus carry (or express) different proteins on the surface of the viral envelope or coat. Influenza is considered a tricky virus because of its ability to change the proteins on its coat. Even subtle changes increase influenza's ability to invade the human body and to cause illness. Antibodies directed against one specific strain of influenza are actually specific against that particular strain's envelope proteins. The body thus needs to produce specific antibodies against different influenza virus envelope proteins in order to effectively

Table 50 Who Should Receive Influenza Vaccination?

Indications for Yearly Seasonal Influenza Vaccination

Vaccination is the best way to prevent illness from influenza.*
Asthma is an indication for influenza vaccination because asthma is considered a
"chronic lung condition" and it complicates the course of illness with influenza.
**In February 2010, the CDC's Advisory Committee on Immunization Practices
(ACIP) recommended "universal influenza vaccination" for all persons, beginning at
6 months of age, beginning in the fall of 2010.**

Vaccination against seasonal influenza is especially recommended for:

- All persons who want to decrease their risk of becoming ill with influenza
- All adults, age 50 and older
- All children and teens, beginning at 6 months of age through 18 years
- All women who are or will be pregnant during influenza season
- Children and teenagers who are receiving long-term aspirin therapy
- Adults and children (6 months of age and older) with a chronic lung or heart condition
- Adults and children (6 months of age and older) with diabetes, chronic blood, kidney, or immune system disease (including that caused by medication, and HIV)
- Adults and children (6 months of age and older) with neurological impairments
- All nursing home or chronic care facility residents
- Persons likely to transmit influenza to others who are at high risk of complications:
  - All healthcare personnel (physicians, nurses, home health aides)
  - Caregivers and household contacts of babies, toddlers, and young children
  - Caregivers and household contacts of adults aged 50 years and older
  - Caregivers and household contacts of persons with high-risk medical conditions, including heart, lung, kidney diseases, and immunosuppressed persons
- Persons who are planning to travel to a part of the world with influenza activity, such as travelers to the tropics, to the Southern hemisphere in April to September, and those who are part of organized tourist groups

A person who has experienced a significant egg allergy, an allergic reaction to a prior influenza vaccination or to any influenza vaccine component, should not receive the influenza vaccine.

Note: The above indications for influenza vaccination apply when vaccine supplies are adequate.
If a vaccine shortage develops, healthy adults younger than 50 years of age should defer vaccination until more vaccine becomes available in order to allow for immunization of persons at higher risk of complications from influenza.

Source: 2009 H1N1 Vaccination Recommendations obtained via the CDC website:
http://www.cdc.gov/h1n1flu/vaccination/acip.htm.

protect against different strains of virus. Antibodies
against one strain are unlikely to offer complete protection
against a different strain that carries a very different coat
or envelope.

Different strains of influenza circulate each flu season, which is why you can get the flu for 2 or more years in succession. It is also the reason that each year, government health agencies advise vaccine manufacturers on what strains to include in that particular year's influenza vaccine. A different influenza vaccine is thus developed and produced each year. The influenza vaccine available each fall in the United States is directed against three specific influenza strains that health authorities believe will cause most of the serious illness during that year's fall and winter influenza season. Each year's vaccine includes one influenza A (H3N2) virus strain, one regular seasonal influenza A (H1N1 type) virus strain (not the 2009 H1N1), and one influenza B virus strain. The vaccine prepared in advance of the 2009 season was thus expected to confer protection against the common disease-causing strains of influenza circulating in the United States during the winter of 2009–2010. The worldwide emergence of illness due to the novel H1N1 in the summer of 2009, after seasonal influenza vaccine production had already begun, mandated that a second vaccine be manufactured to offer protection against that strain, too.

Two types of influenza vaccines are available for prevention of influenza in the United States: the inactivated influenza vaccine, and the live, attenuated influenza vaccine (LAIV) (Table 51). As of this writing, the following five inactivated influenza vaccines are approved for use in the United States: Afluria (manufactured by CSL), Fluarix, FluLaval (both manufactured by GlaxoSmithKline), Fluvirin (manufactured by Novartis), and Fluzone (manufactured by Sanofi Pasteur). Inactivated means that the vaccine contains a killed strain or form of influenza. It is given by injection into a muscle. The inactivated vaccine is the familiar flu shot that has been in clinical use for many years. The LAIV contains a weakened strain of influenza. The LAIV is administered intranasally, by

Table 51   Comparison of Available Seasonal Influenza Vaccines

Inactivated Influenza Vaccine	Live Attenuated Influenza Vaccine

• **The vaccine is recommended for persons with asthma.**
• The vaccine is a "shot" injected into a muscle.
  ○ a thigh muscle in babies aged 6 months to 2 years
  ○ the deltoid muscle in the arm in children >2 years and adults
• The vaccine has been in use for many years.
• The vaccine is approved for children beginning at 6 months of age.
• Children younger than 9 years of age who are getting the vaccine for the first time require two doses of vaccine 4 weeks apart.
• The vaccine contains an inactivated ("killed") form of the virus.
• The vaccine is updated each year.
• The vaccine is best taken each fall, in October or November and is required yearly.
• Protection begins about 14 days after vaccination.
• Protection lasts for about a year.
• Side effects, if any, are usually mild; soreness at the injection site is the most common. Fever and aches can also occur. Call your doctor if you think that you are experiencing a more serious side effect.
	• The vaccine is sprayed into the nostrils.
	• The vaccine was first licensed in the United States in 2003 for use in healthy children and adults from age 2 to 49 years of age.
	• Children between the ages of 2 and 9 years of age who are getting the vaccine for the first time require two doses of vaccine 4 weeks apart.
	• The vaccine contains a live attenuated ("weakened") form of influenza virus.
	• The nasal live attenuated vaccine is not recommended for pregnant women, for children younger than two years of age, for adults older than 50, and is **not recommended for persons with asthma** of any age.
	• The vaccine is updated each year.
	• October or November are the best times for vaccination, which should be repeated yearly.
	• Side effects, if any, are usually mild.
	• Side effects may include runny nose, congestion, cough, mild fever, aches, fatigue, soreness, and in children, abdominal pain, vomiting, or diarrhea. Call your doctor if you think that you are experiencing a more serious side effect.

spraying into the nostrils. The LAIV was first licensed in the United States in 2003. It is manufactured by Wyeth and is named FluMist. Like the inactivated influenza vaccine, LAIV stimulates the body's production of protective antibodies directed against three strains of influenza currently in circulation. Both vaccines are administered each year, ideally in October or November. LAIV, as of this writing, is approved for administration only to healthy persons between ages 2 and 49 years. Unlike the injected inactivated vaccine, LAIV is not approved for use in pregnancy, nor is it approved for persons (of any age) with asthma.

Because influenza can be a fatal and devastating illness, especially in certain groups of individuals, vaccination is recommended for those at high risk of developing medical complications from infection with influenza. *Medical complications* is a term that encompasses hospitalization, severe illness manifestations, respiratory failure, and death. All persons with asthma, including children as well as adults, are candidates for yearly influenza vaccination. Not surprisingly, persons with asthma were also candidates for the 2009 H1N1 inactivated vaccine (Table 52). Only in a few, very specific medical circumstances is vaccination absolutely contraindicated (Table 53). A person who has experienced a significant egg allergy, or an allergic reaction to a prior influenza vaccine or to any constituent

Table 52   Responding to the 2009 H1N1 Influenza Pandemic

In the fall of 2009, a vaccine directed against the H1N1 strain of influenza A virus responsible for a worldwide pandemic influenza was pressed into production. The resultant novel H1N1 vaccine was not a substitute for the seasonal influenza vaccine.

The Centers for Disease Control estimated that approximately 159 million people were candidates for vaccination with the H1N1 vaccine. They include:

- **Pregnant women**—because (1) they are at higher risk of complications and (2) can potentially provide protection to infants who cannot be vaccinated
- **Household contacts and caregivers for children younger than 6 months of age**— because younger infants are at higher risk of influenza-related complications and cannot be vaccinated. Vaccination of those in close contact with infants younger than 6 months old also might help protect infants.
- **Healthcare and emergency medical services personnel**—because infections among healthcare workers can be a potential source of infection for vulnerable patients. Also, increased absenteeism in this population could reduce healthcare system capacity.
- **Children from 6 months through 18 years of age**—because cases of 2009 H1N1 influenza have been seen in children who are in close contact with each other in school and day care settings, which increases the likelihood of disease spread
- **Young adults 19 through 24 years of age**—because many cases of 2009 H1N1 influenza have been seen in these healthy young adults and they often live, work, and study in close proximity, and they are a frequently mobile population;
- **Persons aged 25 through 64 years who have health conditions, including asthma, associated with higher risk of medical complications from influenza.**

Source: 2009 H1N1 Vaccination Recommendations obtained via the CDC Web site: http://www.cdc.gov/h1n1flu/vaccination/acip.htm

Table 53   When to Check With Your Doctor Before Influenza Vaccination

Consult with your physician before obtaining an influenza vaccination if:

- You have a severe allergy to chicken eggs
- You have had an allergic reaction to an influenza vaccination in the past
- You have had an adverse reaction to influenza vaccination in the past
- You have had Guillain-Barré syndrome
- You are currently ill with fever; it is better to wait until you have recovered

of the vaccine should not receive the influenza vaccine. Anyone who has been diagnosed with a neurologic condition called Guillain-Barré syndrome should consult closely with a physician knowledgeable about the risks of vaccination. In general, influenza vaccination is very safe and effective. You cannot get the flu from influenza vaccination, nor can the vaccination cause an infection. It is possible, however, to become ill with influenza even if you received the vaccine, as the vaccine does not protect against all strains of influenza. I remind my patients that the goal of influenza vaccination is to protect them from becoming severely ill from influenza. I still consider vaccination a success if they come down with a milder form of illness that slows them for a few days but does not lead to an exacerbation of their asthma or to hospitalization.

You cannot get the flu from influenza vaccination, nor can the vaccination cause an infection.

82. I am a meticulous housekeeper, so why does my house harbor dust mites? Should people with asthma encase their bedding? Is it a good idea to invest in an air purifier?

Dust mite is a common indoor year-round allergen; allergy to dust mites has been associated with allergic rhinitis and asthma in children, as well as in adults. If you or your child is diagnosed with an allergy to dust mites, your physician will likely advise you on measures you can take to reduce your exposure to dust mites.

Dust mites

Common household allergens. They are microscopic living organisms found indoors in tempered climates, especially in mattresses, bedding, and upholstered furniture.

Dust mites are eight-legged arachnids related to the spider family. Their cast skin and fecal matter are two constituents of house dust to which many people are allergic. The dust mite allergen is concentrated in the mites' fecal droppings. Dust mites live indoors and are present in nearly all homes in areas where the relative humidity is 50% or greater for much of the year. Dust mites are microscopic; you cannot see them without a magnifying microscope. They are so tiny that fifty to seventy dust mites would fit on the head of a pin! They thrive in warm, dark, humid environments, and live off flecks of human skin. They do not drink free water but absorb moisture from the surrounding environment. They can be found in bedding, in upholstered furniture, and in carpeting and draperies. Their presence in your home in no way implies poor housekeeping.

Dust mites cannot survive at a high altitude or in dry environments. Dryer indoor environments with a relative humidity of less than 40% as well as residence at altitude inhibit the growth of dust mites. Could that be why, several generations ago, some persons with asthma whose treatment included a prescription for relocation to the desert or to the mountains had lessening of their symptoms? Was the relocation no more than a move to an area free of dust mite allergen?

Bedding, upholstered couches and chairs, and carpets are areas where dust mites thrive. Ways to reduce your home's dust mite burden include addressing increased levels of humidity if present and removing carpeting and heavy cloth draperies. Consider washable curtains or blinds. Avoid stuffed furniture upholstered with fuzzy fabric. An alternative to removing carpeting involves thorough, daily carpet vacuuming with a high-quality vacuum cleaner, possibly one fitted with a high-efficiency particulate air (HEPA) filter. Steam clean or shampoo carpets and rugs at least once a year. The highest concentration of dust mites in the home usually is found in the bedroom, which thus demands special attention if you or your child is allergic to dust mites. We sleep for hours each night, head on a pillow or two, wrapped up in sheets, blankets and comforters. Since bedding is a favorite location of dust mites, we are, while asleep, in close contact with dust mite antigen, inhaling allergic material all night long. The good news is that there are simple and effective measures you can take to interrupt the replication of dust mites while decreasing the amount of allergen you come into contact with, especially during sleep.

Recommendations for decreasing exposure to dust mites if you or your child is allergic to them begins with the purchase of special dust mite–proof (impervious) encasings for pillows, mattresses, comforters, and box springs. The allergen-impermeable covers are available from retailers specializing in allergy products. If your physician advises you to encase your bedding, make certain the covers you purchase are rated for dust mite protection. Most covers are of high quality and are unobtrusive; you won't even know you're sleeping on one. They usually require washing once a year and carry a warranty for up to 20 years of use. Once you have encased your mattress, box spring, pillows, and comforter, you can further decrease your exposure to dust mite allergen by taking advantage of the fact that dust mites have a life cycle of 2 weeks and cannot survive elevated temperatures. Simply launder sheets, mattress pads, and washable blankets once a week in water heated to a temperature of at least 130°F. The hotter, the better! If the water does not reach at least 130°F (55°C), the dust mites are only getting a bath. Dust mites also set up housekeeping in carpeting

High-efficiency particulate air (HEPA) filter

Filters that meet very stringent filtration requirements. They are capable of trapping particles of very small size, including common indoor allergens, and even certain microorganisms that pose a risk to human health.

Asthma: A Healthy Lifestyle

and in upholstered furniture. If possible, the bedroom should have a wood or tile floor and blinds rather than curtains or drapes. Washable cotton throw rugs can be used in the bedroom to minimize dust mite antigen, provided that you launder the rugs. Stuffed animals or dolls are potential dust mite collectors, and therefore should ideally be kept in a covered toy chest in a room other than the bedroom. Stuffed animals are an abundant source of dust mite allergen, and many children love to collect and sleep with them. Encourage your child to keep the collection in a location other than the bedroom and consider identifying one special stuffed toy to sleep with. Then, if possible, launder the favorite in your washing machine in water hotter than 130°F at least every 2 weeks (every week is best) in order to interrupt the mites' reproductive cycle. Unfortunately, not all stuffed animals are machine washable. Despair not! Plan B involves placing the furry toy in a sealable plastic bag, like a Ziploc bag, sealing it, and placing the bag in your freezer for 12–24 hours once a week.

Should someone with dust mite allergy invest in an air purifier? Be sure to ask your physician or allergist before buying one. Among the options currently available, only a few have been studied in the medical (as opposed to the industrial) literature. Machines that are designed to filter the air in an enclosed space through a fine, HEPA filter are, if used correctly, very efficient in trapping particles of a defined size (usually as small as 0.3 microns). HEPA filters thus reduce the airborne concentration of microscopically small airborne particles, including many aeroallergens, like pollens and dust mites. HEPA-filtering machines must be selected based on the square footage of the enclosed space they will filter. The machines usually contain both a carbon prefilter and a true HEPA filter. The prefilter should be changed every

3–6 months, and the HEPA filter should be replaced every year. HEPA filters are expensive but effective. HEPA filter units do not require much maintenance, apart from filter changes, and they are engineered to run 24 hours a day. They have the disadvantage of being noisy, and they do tend to dry the ambient air. The correct way to run a HEPA unit is to close the room's windows and doors and set the unit's fan on high when you are not home. When you are in the room, at night, for example, set the unit's fan on the highest level you can tolerate from the perspective of noise.

Gemma's comment:

Unfortunately, many standard leases require that three quarters of the floor in every room be carpeted to reduce sound in adjacent apartments, and daily vacuuming is a big task for the housewife with small children. Which is only to say that taking charge of one's asthma is not an easy matter.

83. Is asthma mostly a psychological disease?

No! Asthma is definitely not a psychological disease; it is a physical condition that affects the lungs and its bronchial passages. The concept that asthma is somehow a disease of the mind or an emotional disturbance is false (Table 54). A person experiencing difficulty breathing with cough, increased chest pressure, and wheezing is physically extremely uncomfortable. It is very frightening not to be able to breathe normally and effortlessly, and to instead experience a sensation of oppression. The very real physical discomfort, coupled with the sensations of strenuous breathing, create an extremely unpleasant and very upsetting experience. Until normal, unlabored, and comfortable breathing is reestablished, any person in the midst of an asthma exacerbation feels

Bronchial passages

The breathing tubes of the lungs.

The concept that asthma is somehow a disease of the mind or an emotional disturbance is false.

Table 54   Ten Asthma Myths and Falsehoods

- Having asthma means you have to accept and learn to live with some degree of chest symptoms like cough, uncomfortable breathing, wheezing, and breathlessness.
- Asthma is contagious and can spread to a friend, coworker, classmate, or relative.
- Asthma is all in the mind and only emotionally needy or disturbed persons have asthma.
- Drinking milk and eating dairy products causes mucus production and worsens asthma.
- Mothers with asthma should never breastfeed their infants.
- People with asthma should not exercise.
- Young people with asthma cannot be athletes or participate in competitive sports.
- Children with asthma should be exempted from attending physical education class.
- Persons with asthma will eventually become "dependent" on or "addicted" to their asthma medicines and inhalers with regular use.
- All children with asthma will eventually outgrow the condition and become "cured" over time.

as if they are suffocating. It should come as no surprise that emotions of fear and even panic may occur under these circumstances. These misinterpreted emotional responses are a consequence of the exacerbated asthma symptoms and not the cause of the episode.

The observation that some persons with known asthma develop active symptoms after experiencing very strong emotion, such as shock or grief is another reason why asthma might wrongly be considered a psychological condition. The appropriate strong emotional response acts as a trigger for the development of asthma symptoms and is in no way the underlying cause of the asthma itself. All of us realize that emotional upset can bring on physical symptoms. Some persons develop abdominal discomfort or even heartburn when confronted with a stressful situation, while others may experience a headache in similar circumstances. Similarly, some persons' asthma symptoms may worsen when they confront a situation they experience as stressful. If that is the case, whether it is related to school, family members, coworkers, or others in your circle, it is important that you recognize the potential association between asthma symptoms and harmful stress. Developing working strategies to effectively channel and manage such psychological stress, if present, should include your physician, as it is a component of contemporary comprehensive asthma care.

Gemma's comment:

I've already indicated that, in my experience, with my own asthma and my daughter's, doctors are slow to pick up on asthma symptoms if the patient does not really complain about them. But don't let anyone talk you out of your symptoms or suggest that they are all in your head! Even an educated adult can have a confused reaction to the sense of suffocation that comes with breathlessness, as did one young friend of mine who mistakenly attributed her feeling of panic in the dirty, particle-laden air of a New York City subway to psychological causes. She was starting a new job and, understandably, felt somewhat tense and nervous, but her breathing problems seemed out of line to her, inconsistent with her usual sensible self. After months of worry and seeing several doctors, the diagnosis of asthma really came as a relief and helped her dismiss her fear of a more amorphous, less explicable problem.

PART SEVEN

Special Topic:

Asthma and

Pregnancy

Will pregnancy make my asthma worse?

Can I do anything special during my pregnancy to help protect my unborn child from developing asthma in the future?

Are asthma medications harmful to the unborn child?

Will I be able to breastfeed my baby if I am taking medicine for my asthma?

More . . .

84. Will pregnancy make my asthma worse? How will pregnancy modify or affect my asthma?

Pregnancy will not necessarily make your asthma worse or more symptomatic. Studies of asthma in pregnancy reveal that about one third of pregnant women with asthma will have no change in the degree of their asthma; one third will experience a lessening of their asthma symptoms and a decreased need for medication; and one third will have worsening of the asthma in pregnancy. Approximately one of every three pregnant women with asthma will thus experience more asthma symptomatology and require an increase in asthma medication. After the baby's delivery and the postpartum period, you can expect your asthma to gradually return to usual—whatever the usual was for you!

85. Do I need to see my asthma specialist more frequently now that I am expecting?

Yes, while you are pregnant, you should see your asthma specialist more frequently than before. In my practice, for example, I ask my pregnant patients with asthma to schedule a monthly visit, about as often as they visit the obstetrician. Some women may require more frequent appointments, and some less.

Now that you are pregnant, you and your asthma doctor have an extra point to think about and to take into consideration. The special extra concern is, of course, the health and well-being of the developing fetus. One of the goals of prenatal care for mother and child is the maintenance of a healthy pregnancy to term. Term refers to the time at which the pregnancy is sufficiently advanced to permit the birth of a healthy, fully developed infant, and is defined as anytime after 37 weeks of gestation. A baby's due date is calculated so that it falls exactly 40 weeks after the first day of the mother's last menstrual period. The developing infant is carried in the mother's uterus (or womb). The intrauterine environment is an ideal environment for the fetus, with controlled temperature, oxygen, nutrients, and stimuli. The fetus's oxygen is supplied via the mother's bloodstream through the placenta. The mother's blood oxygen, in turn, reflects her lung function. The overriding principle of asthma treatment in pregnancy is the provision of adequate oxygen to the developing fetus by careful yet aggressive treatment of maternal asthma. The risks of uncontrolled asthma to the mother and infant are far greater than the possible or potential risks of prescribed medication.

The outcome of pregnancy for a woman who has well-controlled asthma can be expected to be no different from the outcome of a woman without asthma. The emphasis is on well-controlled asthma. The goals of asthma treatment in pregnancy parallel those of asthma treatment in general (Table 55). Adherence to prescribed medication is emphasized along with continued lung function and symptom monitoring. Avoidance of known asthma triggers is encouraged as much as possible. Influenza vaccination, as mentioned in Question 81, is recommended for pregnant women who have no contraindication to the vaccine, especially for those who will be in their third trimester of pregnancy during the fall and winter influenza season. Influenza vaccination is safe in pregnancy. The vaccine should not be administered if the patient is allergic to eggs or is allergic to any of the constituents of the vaccine.

Gestation

Another word for pregnancy, gestation is derived from the Latin verb gestare, which means to carry.

The outcome of pregnancy for a woman who has well-controlled asthma can be expected to be no different from the outcome of a woman without asthma.

Special Topic: Asthma and Pregnancy

Table 55   Asthma and Pregnancy: Key Points

- In pregnancy, about one third of women with asthma experience a worsening of their asthma and an increased medication requirement, another third have no significant change in their asthma, and about one third have asthma that is less symptomatic or improved.
- Most asthma exacerbations in pregnancy tend to occur between the 24th and the 36th weeks of pregnancy.
- Flares are rare during the last 4 weeks of pregnancy, and during labor and delivery.
- Poorly controlled asthma in pregnancy is associated with potentially serious complications for both mother and baby, including:
  - Dangerous maternal blood pressure changes (preeclampsia)
  - Premature birth
  - Intrauterine growth retardation
  - Low birth weight
- Uncontrolled asthma in pregnancy poses a greater risk to mother and fetus than any medicine indicated in asthma treatment.
- Well-controlled asthma in pregnancy does not place the mother or infant at increased risk.
- Asthma treatment goals in pregnancy include:
  - Avoidance of asthma triggers (allergic and non-allergic)
  - Absence of asthma symptoms, without restricted activity
  - Restful sleep, uninterrupted by any asthma symptoms
  - Optimized peak flow (PEF) and lung function (FEV_1) measurements
  - Adherence to prescribed asthma medicines
  - Avoidance of cigarette smoke (both maternal smoking and "passive or secondhand")
  - Influenza vaccination for women (who have no absolute contraindication to the vaccine)

86. Can I do anything special during my pregnancy to help protect my unborn child from developing asthma in the future?

The fact that you have asthma does not necessarily mean that your child will develop asthma too. Your asthma diagnosis does, however, place your son or daughter at higher statistical risk of inheriting asthma as compared to a child born to parents with no personal history of asthma. Although there are no specific actions that you can take while pregnant to guarantee that your baby will never develop asthma, many specialists will recommend measures that may possibly delay the onset of allergy and asthma.

The most important steps for you to take while pregnant involve taking excellent care of yourself and making sure that your asthma is well controlled, and hopefully, completely asymptomatic. Studies have shown a link between a mother's lung function and healthier babies at birth. Better maternal lung function leads to improved fetal outcomes, with fewer premature births and fewer complications for the infant. If you are a smoker, smoking cessation is crucial. Pregnancy is an ideal time to quit, for the health of the developing baby, for your health, and for your child's future well-being. Smoking can precipitate an exacerbation of asthma in the mother, and smokers' babies tend to be small, with low birth weights. Children born of mothers who smoke during their pregnancy have an increased incidence of wheezing in infancy. Infants are three times more likely to die of sudden infant death syndrome (SIDS) if their mother smoked during or after pregnancy. There is strong evidence that the children of women who smoked during pregnancy face increased risk for poor lung health as they grow up. Children raised in smokers' homes experience more childhood respiratory illnesses and are at increased risk for the development of asthma. As adults, they even carry an increased risk of certain types of lung cancer—as do the parents who are the active smokers. A child raised in a home with smoking parents is much more likely to become a smoker, as compared to children raised in homes where adults do not smoke.

If you do not smoke, you should avoid exposure to secondhand smoke. Drinking alcoholic beverages in pregnancy is not advised, especially since alcohol contains "empty" (non-nutritive) calories and has adverse effects on the developing fetus. When you plan your meals, limit your intake of the more highly allergenic foods (such as tree nuts, peanuts, shellfish, eggs, and dairy products) as their absence in the maternal diet seems to

Incidence

In medicine, refers to the number of new cases of a disease at any point in time.

Children raised in smokers' homes experience more childhood respiratory illnesses and are at increased risk for the development of asthma.

Special Topic: Asthma and Pregnancy

239

delay the onset of allergy symptoms in a young child. Consider breastfeeding your baby for at least the first 3, and preferably 6, months of his or her life. Breast milk has been shown to support and stimulate the development of your child's immune system. Finally, arrange for prenatal care beginning as early as possible in your pregnancy as it will help provide your newborn child with the best possible health at birth.

87. Are asthma medications harmful to my unborn child?

Studies have been carried out all over the world to help doctors decide which asthma medicines are safest in pregnancy. The single biggest risk to an asthmatic woman's pregnancy is poor asthma control in the mother. Uncontrolled asthma is very harmful to the developing baby and can result in devastating complications for both mother and child. Complications of poorly controlled asthma include pregnancy-induced hypertension, preeclampsia and eclampsia in the mother, preterm labor and premature birth, intrauterine growth retardation, and low-birth-weight babies, along with increased perinatal morbidity and mortality. Inadequate control of the mother's asthma leads to a reduced oxygen supply to the developing baby (maternal hypoxia), as well as a decreased blood supply to the womb. All pulmonary specialists agree that they should treat their pregnant asthma patients with asthma medicines that are not only highly effective, but also as safe as possible for both mother and baby.

Uncontrolled asthma is very harmful to the developing baby and can result in devastating complications for both mother and child.

Hypoxia

Decreased and abnormally low levels of oxygen in the bloodstream.

The FDA classifies all medicines approved since 1980 into one of five different categories. The FDA classification is based on studies of safety in pregnancy. The five categories are A, B, C, D, and X (Table 56). Category A is considered the very safest, while Category X drugs

Table 56   The FDA's Classification of Medicines in Pregnancy

Category	Description
Category A	Adequate and well-controlled studies in pregnant women have not shown an increased risk of fetal abnormalities. ⇒ *Controlled studies show no risk.*
Category B	Animal studies have revealed no evidence of harm to the fetus, but there are no adequate and well-controlled studies in pregnant women. Or . . . Studies in animals have shown an adverse effect on the animal fetus but adequate and well-controlled studies in pregnant women have failed to demonstrate a risk to the human fetus. ⇒ *No evidence of risk in humans.*
Category C	Studies in animals have shown an adverse effect on the animal fetus and there are no adequate and well-controlled studies in pregnant women to assess risk to the human fetus. Or . . . No animal studies of the medicine have been performed and there are no adequate and well-controlled studies in pregnant women to assess risk to the human fetus. ⇒ *Risk cannot be ruled out.*
Category D	Studies, adequate and well-controlled or observational, have demonstrated a risk to the fetus. ***Benefits of therapy with this category of medicine in pregnancy may outweigh the potential risk to the fetus.*** ⇒ *Positive evidence of risk.*
Category X	Studies, adequate and well-controlled or observational, in animals or humans have demonstrated positive evidence of *fetal abnormalities.* ***The use of the medicine is contraindicated in women who are pregnant or who may become pregnant.*** ⇒ *Contraindicated in pregnancy.*

Source: Adapted from: http://www.perinatology.com/exposures/Drugs/FDACategories.htm;
1. FDA Consumer magazine Volume 35, Number 3 May-June 2001.

2. *Physician's Desk Reference.* 57th ed. Montvale, NJ: Thomson PDR; 2004: 3539.

3. Briggs GG, Freeman RK, Yaffe SJ. *Drugs in Pregnancy and Lactation.* 6th ed. Baltimore, MD: Williams & Wilkins, 2002.

are absolutely contraindicated in pregnancy under any circumstances. No medications are labeled Category A for use in pregnancy, because the *A* designation would indicate that relevant drug studies were performed in pregnant women and no such studies have ever been carried out. The safest medicines for practical purposes are labeled as Category B, based on anecdotal reporting involving long-term use in pregnant women and extensive studies (involving pregnant laboratory animals) that produced no evidence of harmful side effects. A Category C designation indicates that the drug has been responsible for some adverse effect on the fetus in animal studies. Drugs in the C category may perhaps carry an increased potential developmental risk to the human fetus, but they are still considered safe for use in pregnant women in part because the dose of medicine used in these animal studies is far, far greater than would ever be given to a human. The decision to use a medication in Category C is determined on a case-by-case basis, most often when the clinical situation is such that the potential risk of not using a Category C medication is greater than the possible risk associated with taking the drug.

There are no asthma medicines classified as Category A, as mentioned previously. Most medicines used in asthma treatment fall into Category C, and several are classified in Category B. All quick-relief, short-acting β_2 agonist inhaled bronchodilator medications (SABA) are classified as Category C, even though they have been in use for over 2 decades and are widely viewed as very safe by the medical profession. All long-acting β_2 agonist inhaled bronchodilators (LABA) are also Category C medicines. The inhaled β_2 agonist medicines have not been shown to have adverse effects on the course of the pregnancy, and have not been shown to be harmful to the human fetus. The *C* classification for the β_2 agonist group of inhalers reflects the absence of studies in pregnant women. One inhaled corticosteroid preparation, Pulmicort (budesonide), is in Category B; all other inhaled steroids are, as of this writing, labeled Category C. The daily use, long-term inhaled controller medicines Intal (cromolyn) and Tilade (nedocromil) are in Category B, as are the leukotriene modifier tablets Singulair (montelukast sodium) and Acolate (zafirlukast). The new IgE blocker Xolair (omalizumab) carries a Category B rating. The theophylline medicines are all Category C drugs.

Because both uncontrolled asthma and poorly controlled asthma in the mother have such serious consequences for her and for her unborn child, the guiding principle in the treatment of asthma in pregnancy is to achieve optimal asthma control even if daily medication is required. It is crucial to normalize maternal lung function and ensure that the mother is not experiencing any symptoms of asthma. Pulmonologists take the point of view that any medicine that is required for best asthma treatment should be administered to a pregnant woman. For example, steroid bursts for treatment of an exacerbation are used in the setting of pregnancy just as they are when a woman is not pregnant. As a rule of thumb, we would use Category B medicines first, adding any required medicines that may fall into the C category (or even D), if needed to achieve good asthma control. If you are pregnant and have any questions or any concerns about the safety of the medicines you have been prescribed, you should consult with your treating physicians. Both your obstetrician and your asthma doctor have the expertise to counsel you and give advice that is best for you. Under no circumstances should you stop your prescribed asthma regimen or not follow the treatment plans recommended by your doctor.

The guiding principle in the treatment of asthma in pregnancy is to achieve optimal asthma control even if daily medication is required.

88. Will I be able to breastfeed my baby if I'm taking medicine for my asthma?

Asthma medicine, especially that administered in inhaled form, is not a contraindication to nursing your infant.

Yes, you will certainly be able to breastfeed if you wish to. Asthma medicine, especially that administered in inhaled form, is not a contraindication to nursing your infant. Breast-feeding has many advantages for both mother and child and may even have beneficial effects in delaying or perhaps avoiding altogether the development of asthma in young children. An Australian study involving over 2000 children found that infants who were exclusively breast-fed, that is, who received only mother's milk for at least the first 4 months of life, had a significantly reduced risk of developing asthma by the age of 6. Breastfeeding also appears to delay the development of allergy in children. Studies indicate that breast-fed children known to be at increased risk for the development of allergy (because of a family history) develop allergies at an older age as compared to children with similar risk factors who are not exclusively breast-fed. Of course, once your baby is born, you should seek guidance from the pediatrician if you are taking any over-the-counter or prescription medicines in addition to your asthma medicine while you are breastfeeding.

PART EIGHT

Special Topic: Asthma in Children

Can I catch asthma from my child who has asthma?

Do milk products cause increased mucus in persons who have asthma, especially children?

Should I take my four-year-old to a physician who specializes in asthma? Can the primary care pediatrician diagnose and treat her asthma?

Will my child outgrow his asthma?

How can I help my son's school staff cope with his asthma and know how to handle an emergency?

Our 10-year-old daughter who has asthma wants to go to sleep-away camp next summer. Should she attend a regular camp or a camp for children with asthma?

More . . .

89. Can I catch asthma from my child who has asthma?

Asthma is not an infectious condition. It cannot be transmitted from person to person, nor can it spread between people.

Absolutely not! Asthma is not an infectious condition. It cannot be transmitted from person to person, nor can it spread between people. Remember that there is an inherited component to the development of asthma and it is well established that the tendency to develop asthma runs in families. If one parent has asthma or certain allergies, a child has a greater chance of developing asthma and/or allergies than does a child of unaffected parents, who have neither asthma nor allergies. The chance of a child developing asthma increases further when both parents have asthma. The exact role of genetics and the inheritance patterns of asthma are not well understood, and genetic inheritance alone is far from the whole story. Environmental factors clearly play a role in asthma development. If your child has asthma, and you are later diagnosed with asthma, too, this does not mean that you somehow "caught" asthma from your child; rather, your asthma diagnosis reflects genetic and environmental factors common to both you and your child.

90. Do more boys than girls have asthma?

As young children, boys are almost twice as likely as girls are to develop asthma.

Yes, but only as children. As young children, boys are almost twice as likely as girls are to develop asthma. Interestingly, the pattern is reversed when looking at asthma in older age groups. An article published in the medical journal *Chest* in October 2003 found that 62% of children with asthma (asthma patients younger than 18 years of age) were male, while 68% of the adult patients with asthma were female. In studies of severe asthma, the preponderance of boys is notable as well: 2 of 3 children with severe asthma are boys. But, among adults with severe asthma, women account for two thirds of those affected. The gender-based differences are not understood. Theories suggest the influence of female hormones, as well as the difference in size between male and female lungs as they grow into adulthood.

Kerrin's comment:

I find it interesting that my daughter never suffered from any allergies or asthma, but that my son has been struggling with both since shortly after he was born. After hearing all of the theories as to why this might be, a few pieces seem to fit into the puzzle. Besides the greater tendency for young boys to develop asthma than young girls, my daughter began going to day care in the first year of her life. Of course, when she first started going, she would get sick a lot. Eventually, however, she seemed to adjust to the increased exposure to germs and would only very occasionally get sick. My son didn't start going to day care until after he was 2 years old, and is still very sensitive to germs, becoming sick on an almost weekly basis, with his asthma symptoms kicking in every time.

91. If my 7-year-old daughter wheezes, does it mean that she has asthma?

Maybe not, but asthma is very likely. Repeated bouts of wheezing in school-aged children—boys and girls—are almost always caused by asthma. The likelihood of asthma is even greater when a cough accompanies wheezing. A family history of asthma or allergy is an important risk factor for the development of asthma. Not all children who wheeze, however, have asthma. Medical evaluation of a child who is wheezing must include consideration of other possible causes for the wheeze in order to establish the diagnosis (Table 57). The list of such possibilities is called the differential diagnosis. Causes of wheezing in children include congenital abnormalities, such as tracheal webs; various types of infections; tumors; cardiac conditions; and other illnesses, such as cystic fibrosis.

Differential diagnosis

The process of considering different conditions or diseases that could be responsible for a patient's symptoms. After reviewing the patient's history, findings of the physical examination, and laboratory and test data, a physician will generate a list of differential diagnoses.

Cystic fibrosis

A congenital metabolic disorder that primarily involves the lungs and the gastrointestinal system.

Table 57   Causes of Wheezing in Children

Wheeze is a major symptom of asthma and children with recurrent episodes of wheezing likely have asthma. Not all children who wheeze however have asthma.

Conditions other than asthma that may cause wheezing in children include:

- Anatomic abnormalities
  - Bronchopulmonary dysplasia
  - Hypertrophy of tonsils and/or adenoids
  - Primary ciliary dyskinesia
  - Retrognathia (Pierre-Robin syndrome)
  - Tracheal stenosis
  - Tracheo-bronchomalacia
  - Vascular rings
- Cardiomegaly (enlarged heart)
- Cystic fibrosis
- Foreign body aspiration
- Gastroesophageal reflux (GERD)
- Infections of the lung, epiglottis, tonsillar area
  - Bronchiolitis
  - Bronchitis
  - Epiglottitis
  - Peritonsillar abscess
  - Retropharyngeal abscess
  - Tracheitis (bacterial)
- Tumors
- Vocal cord dysfunction (VCD) syndrome

Asthma is often underdiagnosed or missed in children.

Asthma is often underdiagnosed or missed in children. As any parent knows, children frequently catch many colds each year, especially when school is in session. Some children with undiagnosed asthma are erroneously thought to have recurrent chest infections when they in fact have asthma. It is important for physicians to distinguish asthma from repeated episodes of bronchitis and infections, such as pneumonia. Do not assume that your child is experiencing a "bad winter" if she seems to be getting chest cold after chest cold; she may have asthma (Table 58). If so, make sure that she gets appropriate

Table 58   Is My Child's Diagnosis Asthma?

The diagnosis of asthma in a child is more likely when certain symptoms are present. The diagnosis may be less straightforward in a child with atypical symptoms.

Important symptoms to report to and review with your child's doctor include:

- The presence of **wheezing** including any pattern of presentation and the identification of any particular obvious precipitating causes.
- The presence of **cough** and its nature (such as wet, dry, and/or productive) and the situations that appear to cause this symptom, such as exposure to certain environments (for example: near pets, when in a smoke filled restaurant, or around strong perfumes) at certain seasons of the year (for example: in the spring).
- Abnormal and/or uncomfortable sensations of breathing or, in medical terms, **dyspnea**.
- Occurrence of episodic **chest tightness or pressure**.
- Decrease in **exercise tolerance**, which limits participation in exercise or sports.
- **Nighttime chest symptoms** such as cough, wheeze, and/or chest tightness that awaken your child from sleep.
- Lingering "colds" that "always go to the chest" and last more than 10 days or so.

In addition to evaluating your child's symptoms, the physician will consider additional data:

- Past medical and family history: any personal or family history of asthma, allergy, or conditions such as eczema or hay fever.
- Results of specialized testing such as:
  - Pulmonary function tests (PFTs) with FEV_1
  - Peak expiratory flow (PEF) monitoring
  - Chest X-rays (may occasionally be required)
  - Allergy testing, either directly (prick/puncture or intradermal skin testing) or indirectly (by a blood [RAST/ImmunoCAP] test).

medical care to establish an accurate diagnosis and receive correct treatment.

92. Do milk products cause increased mucus in persons who have asthma, especially children?

Milk is not a cause of increased mucus production, nor is it considered to be an asthma trigger (see Table 21). Consumption of milk has no effect on lung capacity, either deleterious or beneficial. It is a myth that milk is somehow harmful to children with asthma. A recent

It is a myth that milk is somehow harmful to children with asthma.

study on the effects of milk consumption in asthma performed by Brunello Wüthrich, MD, Alexandra Schmid, Barbara Walther, PhD, and Robert Sieber, PhD, and published in the December 2005 issue of *The Journal of the American College of Nutrition* concludes:

> *People with asthma are sometimes advised to abstain from the consumption of dairy products, but research shows that consumption of milk does not significantly change various lung function parameters . . . Recommendations to abstain from dairy products due to the belief that they induce symptoms of asthma are not supported by the body of research evidence on the relationship between dairy consumption and occurrence of asthma. Furthermore, in general, there is no evidence to explain an underlying mechanism linking dairy and asthma. Therefore, people with asthma do not need to avoid the consumption of dairy products to control symptoms.*

Vitamin

A substance required in minute quantities for health. Vitamins occur naturally in a wide range of foods. Vitamin deficiencies are unusual in Western society, and they reflect either a disease of the absorptive capacity of the gastrointestinal system with consequent malabsorption of nutrients or a severely restricted diet.

Milk can, however, be an allergen in sensitized children. Cow's milk allergy is a true food allergy and is due to an allergy to the protein constituents of the milk. Like many food allergies, milk allergy usually manifests as gastrointestinal symptoms or as a skin reaction such as hives or eczema, as a runny nose, but not as increased mucus. If you suspect that milk does not agree with your child, bring it to your physician's attention. Do not automatically eliminate milk and milk products from the child's diet without medical consultation and advice.

Growing children need calcium in their diets to promote bone health and proper development. In addition to calcium, dairy products are a significant dietary source of several other important nutrients, including protein, riboflavin, and vitamins A and B_{12}. You should consider having your child evaluated for possible milk allergy if you have any concerns about milk and dairy products affecting their asthma. If your child is allergic to milk, treatment will include elimination of dairy products. Your physician will assist you in modifying your child's diet without compromising his or her nutritional status.

93. The pediatrician says that my toddler has a "wheezy chest" but that asthma cannot be diagnosed until my son is older than 2 or even 3 years old. Why is that?

The observation that your young son is wheezing does not necessarily mean that he has asthma. Wheezing in infancy is never normal and should be reported to the pediatrician. Many children do wheeze during their first 12 months of life and only a small percentage of them ultimately develop asthma over time. The major stimulus to wheezing in the toddler years is typically a viral respiratory tract infection.

Wheezing in infancy is never normal.

Wheezing in very young children is categorized into two general patterns: non-allergic wheezing and allergic wheezing (Table 59). In the first instance, wheezing

The major stimulus to wheezing in the toddler years is typically a viral respiratory tract infection.

Table 59   Patterns of Wheezing in Infants and Babies

Non-Allergic Wheezing Pattern

- Wheezing typically occurs in the setting of a viral upper respiratory tract infection.
- Eczema, allergic rhinitis, and food allergy are not usually present.
- Wheezing abates as the baby grows and reaches preschool age (ages 3–6).
- The wheezing seen in infancy in these children is *not* a harbinger of asthma.

Allergic Wheezing Pattern

- Wheezing typically occurs in the setting of a viral upper respiratory tract infection.
- Maternal allergy or asthma is often present.
- Eczema, allergic rhinitis, and food allergy are typically also present.
- As the child grows, the pattern of wheezing when the child is ill with upper respiratory viral infections continues.
- The wheezing seen in infancy in these children is likely a symptom of asthma, which potentially persists over time.

occurs when the infant becomes ill with an acute upper respiratory viral infection. The child's airways grow larger in the preschool years, and the wheezing disappears as the toddler grows. In non-allergic wheezing, symptoms seen in infancy do not recur with subsequent upper respiratory viral infections. The "wheezy chest" is not an early manifestation of asthma.

Infants who exhibit the second, allergic, pattern also wheeze when infected with an acute upper respiratory virus. However, they are more likely to have real asthma that continues throughout childhood. They are also more likely to have diagnosed allergies such as allergic rhinitis, food allergy, or eczema. Their airways will also grow larger as they become toddlers, but the wheezing persists. They have asthma, not a narrowed, immature airway as a cause of wheezing in infancy during upper respiratory viral infections.

It is difficult for doctors to be certain that a child has asthma or has allergic wheezing, before the age of 18–24 months. This is not to say that children younger than that do not develop asthma, only that it is not easy to confidently make a definitive diagnosis at that time. For practical purposes, the diagnosis of bronchial asthma in a very young child is generally based on a recurring pattern of cough and/or wheeze that responds to a bronchodilator short term and that is further controlled long term with anti-inflammatory medication. A definitive diagnosis of asthma is also more likely in children under the age of 3 years if the child has experienced more than three episodes of wheezing in the prior 12 months, if the child has a confirmed diagnosis of eczema (atopic dermatitis) and/or allergic rhinitis, if there is a parental history of asthma, and if wheezing has occurred in the absence of a cold or infection.

Kerrin's comment:

I recall being very frustrated by the fact that no one would or could diagnose my son with asthma with certainty before he was about 2 years old. Only after he had three episodes of respiratory difficulty did I hear the word asthma *mentioned with conviction. As a parent, you want to know exactly what is happening with your child so that you can be educated and prepared, but without a definite diagnosis of anything, I constantly felt very anxious about his health. After he was finally diagnosed, we were able to educate ourselves about the condition and begin preventive treatment plans. My son was prescribed Zyrtec [cetirizine] at the same time he was officially diagnosed with asthma. He takes it every day, along with Singulair [montelukast]. His asthma symptoms have been well controlled since he started taking these medications, and his allergies have also been manageable.*

94. Should I take my 4-year-old to a physician who specializes in asthma? Can the primary care pediatrician diagnose and treat her asthma?

Of the nearly 7 million children with asthma in the United States, the majority are diagnosed and initially treated by their primary care physician. If your child's asthma is mild in severity and well controlled, there may be no reason to see an asthma specialist, pulmonologist, or allergist. The key phrase in the last sentence is *well controlled*. According to the guidelines established by the National Asthma Education and Prevention Program (NAEPP), asthma control has been achieved when your child has no coughing, no difficulty in breathing, no nighttime awakening because of cough or wheeze, no acute asthma episodes, no absences from school or activities, and the parent or caregiver has not missed time from work due to the child's asthma. Objectively, your child should have normal or near-normal lung function. If these criteria are fulfilled, your child's asthma is well controlled.

You should arrange for your child to see an asthma specialist if your child's asthma is active for most days, if there are frequent nighttime asthma symptoms that interfere with sleep and rest, if your child is absent from preschool because of asthma symptoms, or if your child requires hospital emergency room visits for asthma. You should also consider seeking a consultation with an asthma expert if you (or your older child) believe that asthma symptoms are not controllable, or if you do not understand how to take care of those symptoms. You might seek consultation from either a pediatric pulmonologist or from a pediatric allergist. After your child has undergone the appropriate evaluation, you and the specialist can decide whether the child requires continuing ongoing care from an asthma specialist or if your pediatrician can resume caring for your child's asthma.

The most recent 2007 update of the NAEPP's *Expert Panel Report* addresses the question of when infants and children 5 years of age or younger should be referred to an asthma specialist and when children aged 5 to 11 should be referred. You should bring your child to an asthma specialist if your child has experienced an asthma exacerbation requiring hospitalization (inpatient care) and/or if therapy with either omalizumab or immunotherapy (allergy shots) is being considered. Consultation with an asthma specialist is also recommended for all young children with moderate or severe persistent asthma. Similarly, referral to an asthma specialist should be considered for infants and very young children with mild persistent asthma.

Gemma's comment:

Yes! The focused attention of both physician and patient is all-important. During her early years, my daughter's allergies and asthma symptoms were repeatedly overlooked by the busy pediatricians who saw her only for a few overbooked minutes in a crowded office full of crying babies and frazzled moms.

95. Will my child outgrow his asthma?

Asthma is never outgrown. Asthma is a lifelong diagnosis. Symptoms of asthma, however, can become absent for long periods of time, on the order of years in many cases, and thus lead to the impression that a child has outgrown the disease. The state of baseline hyperreactivity (discussed in Question 12) that defines asthma never disappears. Many boys and girls who have asthma during their early childhood years do indeed become symptom-free as adolescents, and even beyond. It is easy to then erroneously equate the disappearance of asthma symptoms over time with "outgrowing" asthma. Contemporary medical thinking views the phenomenon of disappearing asthma as a state of very prolonged asthma remission during which symptoms abate. Although epidemiologic studies do confirm the phenomenon, too many general pediatricians falsely reassure parents that their child will "outgrow" their asthma symptoms and the need for asthma medication by young adulthood. The reason may be partly related to the doctor's personal clinical experience of treating youngsters with asthma. As you can easily imagine, a 34-year-old father of two, who begins to wheeze again for the first time since he was 14 years old, generally does not call his former pediatrician to report this medical development!

If you ask an asthma specialist if your son's asthma symptoms will decrease, increase, or disappear with the passage

Asthma is never outgrown. Asthma is a lifelong diagnosis.

of time, a realistic response might be, "I don't know, since I cannot predict in advance what will happen to your particular child's asthma." Certain clinical clues do appear to indicate a greater likelihood of asthma symptoms decreasing over time. There seems to be a greater likelihood that a child will stop experiencing asthma symptoms with the passage of time if they have no parental history of asthma and allergy, if their symptoms of cough or wheezing began early in life, and if their primary trigger was a respiratory tract infection. Many children with these characteristics are free of asthma symptoms within the first decade of life. Ongoing symptomatic asthma requiring medicine has on the other hand, been associated with the presence of clinical symptoms of both asthma and eczema; wheezing that develops in the absence of infection; older age of symptom onset; asthma and/or allergy in the parents, especially the mother; and physician-diagnosed allergic rhinitis in a child who has experienced previous episodes of asthma.

Although we all have a tendency to want information on what to expect or on what lies ahead, particularly for our children and their health, there is no way to accurately predict the course of asthma symptoms in any individual over time. The results of studies, as described above, may help your child's doctor hazard an educated guess, but my perspective is to instead refocus on the present and obtain the best asthma care for your child. Learn about asthma—reading this book is, of course, an excellent step in that regard—and ensure that your child's asthma is controlled through adherence to a comprehensive asthma treatment plan. We all want our children to be as healthy as they can possibly be, and we want them to grow into happy and fulfilled adults. Well-controlled asthma is not a barrier to any of those goals!

96. Should my child be excused from physical education classes since she's been diagnosed with asthma?

No, absolutely not. Your child's asthma should be brought under good control, and then she should be encouraged to participate fully in all aspects of school life, including fitness and sports. A diagnosis of asthma should never automatically lead to curtailed physical activity. Participation in physical education and in team sports is an important component of the healthy lifestyle advocated for all persons with asthma. Having your child excused from physical education class not only robs her of the benefits associated with exercise, but also stigmatizes her and sends the wrong message that asthma is an insurmountable physical impairment.

97. How can I help my son's school staff cope with his asthma and know how to handle an emergency?

The best way to make sure that your son's school is in a position to handle his asthma is to continue to teach him about his asthma and the medicines he takes and to establish effective communication with all of his teachers and the school nurse. Your son's ability to recognize and act on his asthma symptoms will, of course, evolve depending on his age and maturity. Even though asthma is a common condition throughout childhood and adolescence, it is still a good idea to make sure that school staff knows about your son's asthma. The adage, "Never assume" applies! You should meet with your son's teacher and possibly the nurse (if there is one) early in the school year to discuss his medical history. It would be appropriate to have a list of the daily medications that he takes as well as those, such as quick-relief bronchodilator MDIs (albuterol) that should be administered to treat an acute symptom or exacerbation.

The updated 2007 NAEPP *Expert Panel Report* (*EPR-3*) recommends that physicians caring for children with asthma prepare an individualized written asthma action plan for each child that is specifically designed for school or the child care setting. It further specifies that each school action plan contain instructions for handling exacerbations (including the doctor's recommendation regarding student self-administration of medication); recommendations for daily use, long-term control medications and for the prevention of exercise-induced bronchospasm (EIB), if appropriate; and identification of those factors that make the student's asthma worse, so the school may help the student avoid exposure. The NHLBI offers written resources for schools and school staff on its Web site addressing all aspects of asthma management in schools—see http://www.nhlbi.nih.gov/health/prof/lung/ index.htm. You can also view several sample asthma action plans online by typing "school asthma action plan" in your browser. The Asthma and Allergy Foundation of America has a sample student asthma card on its Web site. You can view it online (http://www.aafa.org).

You should familiarize yourself with the school district's policies (if any) regarding the use of asthma medication in the school setting. Some schools allow students to carry their quick-relief bronchodilator inhaler with them at all times, whereas others require that it be left in the school nurse's office. The former is obviously far more desirable than the latter. I insist that my patients carry their inhaled bronchodilator with them throughout the school day. The NAEPP and other authorities advocate that students with asthma be allowed to carry their asthma medicine (especially an inhaled quick-relief bronchodilator or SABA) for self-administration as required during the school day, with prior parental and physician okay of course! Several states have enacted legislation to allow students to carry their asthma medicine at all times during the school day. That policy is especially appropriate for student athletes with EIB who require pre-medication with bronchodilator medicine before exercise. Make sure to review any of your concerns with your son's doctor in advance of the school year; a good time might be when the physician fills out the required pre-enrollment health forms. The school should be given a written copy of the action plan, treatment plan, and your son's medication list. Make sure that your son learns when and how to use his quick-relief inhaler. If he is old enough, he should also learn, just to be on the safe side, the correct technique for using an MDI without a valved holding chamber (VHC) even though he usually would use an MDI and VHC together. You may also consult several very useful, patient-centered asthma Web sites mentioned in Appendix 1 for additional pointers.

Valved holding chamber (VHC)

A device that facilitates the inhalation of medicine from a metered-dose inhaler (MDI).

Kerrin's comment:

The day care where my son goes has many people who are familiar with how to work the nebulizer. Because allergies and asthma are so prevalent these days, it's not difficult to find people knowledgeable about the condition and treatment. Whenever he has a cold, we send the nebulizer and vials of albuterol to school with him, and one of the teachers administers a treatment before he goes down for a nap and later in the afternoon before I pick him up. This way he is able to get the four treatments per day that his doctor recommends during the times when he is at the greatest risk for having his asthma symptoms triggered.

98. Our 10-year-old daughter who has asthma wants to go to sleep-away camp next summer. Should she attend a regular camp or a camp for children with asthma?

The answer to what type of summer camp might be best for your daughter with asthma depends on several factors. Considerations include the severity of her asthma, her level of asthma control, and importantly, how effectively she copes both practically and emotionally with her asthma symptoms and exacerbations. Like a pendulum, our perspective on camps that are limited to children with a specific medical condition swing back and forth. For a child who has recently been diagnosed with asthma, being in an environment where all the children have the same condition can be very positive. Your child will learn that she is not the only one who has to learn to live with asthma. More importantly, the constructive examples of good self-management skills exhibited by other, knowledgeable children with asthma will go a long way toward improving your daughter's appreciation of the fact that she can control her symptoms, thereby increasing her self-image and well-being.

In the unique environment that an asthma camp provides, your child will not only have a good social experience but, equally importantly, will become more confident in her ability to deal with a potential pattern of recurring symptoms. Children who go to an asthma camp become more informed about their disease and therefore may be more effective in taking an active role in self-management. Depending on their age, children will learn how and when to take their medications and become accustomed to the routine of a regular dosing schedule. The time spent at camp can provide an intensive educational experience, which is critical for the development of appropriate asthma self-management skills.

The increased knowledge that comes from attending an asthma camp and the self-confidence your child will develop from realizing that she can control the disease most of the time (rather than the other way around) makes it an invaluable experience. Many children realize, and some for the first time, that they can participate in almost all sports activities. Through age-appropriate teaching, campers will learn why they need to take their medicines. As a direct result of the time spent at camp, most children will have fewer unscheduled asthma visits to their pediatrician and the emergency room upon their return.

Naturally, the ultimate goal for any child with a medical condition is for them to function as normally as possible and to fulfill not only their potential, but also their hopes and dreams. Children who have asthma can accomplish this goal within the framework of an appropriate, comprehensive asthma management plan. Asthma should not compromise your child's ability to perform well at school, on the athletic field, or at home. Time spent at an asthma camp can provide your child with the self-management tools to help make this happen. However, like so many other things, rarely does one size fit all, and therefore not every child who has asthma must go or should go only to an asthma-oriented camp. For some children, a potential problem with going to an asthma camp is that too much attention is focused on the disease and not enough on the other social, educational, and athletic aspects of a camp experience. Others may want to attend the same camp that their schoolmates attend. Many children with asthma have had rewarding camp experiences at regular summer camps. Each child's situation is different; deciding which type of camp will provide the best experience for a particular child is an individual's choice.

You can find a list of asthma camps maintained by the Consortium of Children's Asthma Camps on the Internet at http://www.asthmacamps.org/asthmacamps/findacamp/usmap.asp?topic=parentsandcampers.

99. Will my smoking cigarettes affect my child who has just been diagnosed with asthma?

Yes, your smoking will affect your child with newly diagnosed asthma. Smoking should be categorically banned from any household in which a child has asthma of any severity. Your smoking affects your child in many different ways. Every child today knows that smoking is bad for you. Some are aware of the links between cigarette smoking and lung diseases such as emphysema. Others know about links between smoking and lung and bladder cancers, as well as the fact that cigarette smoking causes heart disease and stroke. Your smoking adversely affects your health and decreases your life expectancy; both factors certainly impact your children. Children of parents who smoke are themselves more likely to become smokers in adolescence and beyond. Your smoking provides a bad model for your child who is much more likely to do as you do rather than do as you say. Children raised in a home where adults smoke have an increased risk of developing asthma.

Your child has just been diagnosed with asthma. Look at it from your son or daughter's perspective. Until the diagnosis was made and medicine prescribed, he or she was experiencing asthma symptoms. To get an idea of what that might be like, try a simple experiment. Get a very narrow straw or plastic coffee stirrer and place it in your mouth. Breathe through the narrow straw (or plastic coffee stirrer) by pinching your nostrils together. Then, march briskly in place. You will become aware of a very uncomfortable sensation of breathing, and it will take a great deal of effort to keep marching in place. The breathing experiment you have just performed approximates how it might feel to breathe through constricted breathing passages.

Your child has been feeling poorly, has undergone a medical evaluation, and now has to take medicine and adapt to his or her new diagnosis. Depending on the child and his or her age, as well as the severity of the asthma, the entire family is entering a period of change and adaptation. As a parent, you may be experiencing increased stress. If you are a smoker, you may crave cigarettes more intensely than usual. Cigarette smoking is a universal asthma trigger. Your continued smoking will contribute to increased symptoms in your child, along with an increased medication requirement. My advice: quit smoking, both for your health and that of your children. Parents who attempt to limit their smoking to the bathroom, garage, or basement are still smoking indoors where the smoke can be trapped and circulated back into the house. Anywhere air can travel, smoke can travel too—and even limited exposure to secondhand smoke is too much for a child with asthma. Parents who smoke in the home are also sending their children the message that their smoking is more important to them than their children's health; this message, unspoken though it may be, can undermine the child's understanding of how important it is to take asthma symptoms seriously and may affect the child's willingness to comply with his or her program of asthma treatment.

100. My child with asthma is also allergic to our family pet. How important is it for us to find a new home for our pet?

It is crucially important that you relocate your pet to a new home. If your child is allergic to the family pet, and especially if the pet allergy is a trigger for your child's asthma, it is in your child's medical best interest for you to relocate the animal. A fundamental principle of allergy control is known as allergen avoidance. After an individual has been diagnosed with a clinical allergy to a specific allergen, the goal of allergen avoidance is the elimination of any and all exposures to that specific allergen. Allergen avoidance, if successful, is a highly effective measure in allergy treatment. Some allergens, such as dust mites or molds, are so ubiquitous that it can be nearly impossible to completely remove them from the home environment. Others, such as pet dander, are far easier to address. If you remove the family pet from your home, and you are then able to rid your home of any pet allergen left behind, your child will likely have a significant lessening in allergy and asthma symptoms, as well as decreased medication requirements.

Although parents understand and comply with the concept of decreasing the level of indoor allergens by controlling dust mites or eliminating roaches, it is an entirely different situation when the family pet is the source of the allergen. When doctors recommend removing a pet from the household, they somehow instantly morph into a kind of enemy or ogre. Unfortunately, many children have significant asthma problems triggered by household pets like cats, dogs, ferrets, rabbits, hamsters, and gerbils. The relationship between a newly acquired pet and your child's asthma (or allergy) symptoms may become obvious very rapidly or may develop more insidiously. A tricky situation arises when an animal has been in the home for months or even years before symptoms appear. Parents and children alike have a difficult time understanding how the child could have lived with a pet for such a long time before developing symptoms. The fact is that the time it takes to become sensitized to any allergen, including a pet, can vary from days to years.

Much to the dismay of allergists, pulmonologists, and pediatricians, most people generally will not relocate a pet who has become a member of the family. Second-best (and we truly mean second-best) recommendations include keeping the animal out of your child's bedroom at all times, even when your child is at school or away from home. Dogs can be trained to avoid certain rooms or areas relatively easily, but with cats—animals notorious for their curiosity and lack of obedience—you and your child must make a habit of keeping the child's room strictly secured from the cat's access at all times. Another measure applies if your home has forced air heating. Make sure that the vents in your child's room are covered with appropriate filters. An allergist can provide you with specific recommendations depending on what type of pet you have and the layout of your home. If your cat or dog will cooperate, a weekly bath will help lower the level of animal allergen in your home. These steps may be helpful, but they are truly a distant second best to not having a pet at all.

Gemma's comment:

Obviously, it's best to relocate your pet or never get one in the first place. But your child may feel very strongly about having a pet, especially in the early school years when show-and-tell sessions often turn on stories about household members, including pets, family trips, etc. I've known nursery school teachers who insist that every child should have a pet (turtles or fish won't do!).

A selective listing of books published since 2003, resources, and references about asthma follows.

If you have any specific clinical question about your asthma in particular, always seek personalized advice from your treating physician.

Books for Children

Abby's Asthma and the Big Race by Theresa Golding and Margeaux Lucas. Albert Whitman & Company, 2009. ISBN-13: 978-0807504659.

I Have Asthma (Let's Talk About It Books) by Jennifer Moore-Mallinos and Marta Fabrega. Barron's Educational Series, 2007. ISBN-13: 978-0764137853.

Peter, the Knight with Asthma by Janna Matthies and Anthony Lewis. Albert Whitman & Company, 2009. ISBN-13: 978-0807565179.

Books for Parents and Teens

100 Questions & Answers About Your Child's Asthma, by Claudia S. Plottel, MD, and B. Robert Feldman, MD. Jones and Bartlett Publishers, 2008. ISBN-13: 978-0763739171.

The Asthma and Allergy Action Plan for Kids: A Complete Program to Help Your Child Live a Full and Active Life by Allen Dozor and Kate Kelly. Fireside, 2004. ISBN-13: 978-0743235778.

Breathe Easy! A Teen's Guide to Allergies and Asthma by Jean Ford. Mason Crest Publishers, 2005. ISBN-13: 978-1590848425.

The Children's Hospital of Philadelphia Guide to Asthma: How to Help Your Child Live a Healthier Life by Julian Lewis Allen, MD, Tyra Bryant-Stephens, MD, and Nicholas A. Pawlowski, MD, with Sheila Buff and Martha M. Jablow. Wiley, 2004. ISBN-13: 978-0471441168.

The Complete Kid's Allergy and Asthma Guide: The Parent's Handbook for Children of All Ages by Milton Gold. Robert Rose Inc., 2003. ISBN-13: 978-0778800781.

Books on Adult Asthma

Asthma for Dummies by William E. Berger. John Wiley & Sons, Inc., 2004. ISBN-13: 978-0764542336.

Harvard Medical School Adult Asthma: Your Guide to Breathing Easier by Christopher H. Fanta. Harvard Medical School, 2007. ISBN-13: 978-1933812281.

The Harvard Medical School Guide to Taking Control of Asthma by Christopher H. Fanta, Kenan Haver, Lynda Cristiano, with Nancy Waring. Free Press, 2003. ISBN-13: 978-0743224789.

Life and Breath: The Breakthrough Guide to the Latest Strategies for Fighting Asthma and Other Respiratory Problems—At Any Age by Neil Schachter. Broadway, 2004. ISBN-13: 978-0767912891.

One-Minute Asthma: What You Need to Know, 8th ed., by Thomas F. Plaut. Pedipress.com, 2008. ISBN-13: 978-0914625308.

What to Do When the Doctor Says It's Asthma by Paul Hannaway. Fair Winds Press, 2004. ISBN-13: 978-1592331048.

Organizations

Allergy and Asthma Network Mothers of Asthmatics, Inc. (AANMA)

2751 Prosperity Avenue, Suite 150, Fairfax, VA 22031

1-800-878-4403

www.aanma.org

Magazine: *Allergy and Asthma Today*

Newsletter: *The MA Report*

The AANMA is a nonprofit, community-based organization founded in 1985 by Nancy Sander, a parent of a child with asthma. The organization publishes several practical booklets on asthma and allergy management. Membership in the network includes a newsletter, magazine, toll-free helpline, and discounts on products.

American Academy of Allergy, Asthma, and Immunology (AAAAI)

611 East Wells Street, Milwaukee, WI 53202

1-800-822-2762

www.aaaai.org

The AAAAI is the largest professional medical specialty organization in the United States representing professionals in the fields of allergy, asthma, and immunology. One of its primary goals is to disseminate cutting-edge information on asthma and allergy to both physicians and the public.

American Academy of Pediatrics (AAP)

141 N.W. Point Boulevard, Elk Grove Village, IL 60007

1-847-434-4000

www.aap.org

This site has an extensive list of current literature on all phases of asthma. A useful source of information for the entire family.

American College of Allergy, Asthma, and Immunology (ACAAI)

85 West Algonquin Road, Suite 550, Arlington Heights, IL 60005

1-800-842-7777

www.acaai.org

The college represents thousands of specially trained physicians in the field of asthma, allergy, and immunology. Educating the public about the state-of-the-art management of allergy and asthma has been one of the organization's primary objectives since its foundation.

American Lung Association (ALA)

61 Broadway, New York, NY 10006

To contact your local chapter, call 1-800-LUNG-USA

www.lungusa.org

Local ALA chapters sponsor the Open Airways for Schools elementary school-based asthma education program. The ALA provides information on asthma camps as well as educational materials, speakers, and resources on asthma for all age groups.

Asthma and Allergy Foundation of America (AAFA)

1233 20th Street NW, Suite 402, Washington, DC 20036

1-800-7ASTHMA

www.aafa.org

Newsletter: *The Asthma and Allergy Advance*

The AAFA is a private, nonprofit organization dedicated to finding a cure for and educating the public about asthma and allergies. AAFA offers community workshops and newsletters for adults and teens with asthma. Their resource catalog is full of educational information for educators, parents, and children.

Food Allergy and Anaphylaxis Network (FAAN)

11781 Lee Jackson Highway, Suite 160, Fairfax, VA 22033-3309

1-800-929-4040

www.foodallergy.org

The FAAN is dedicated to raising public awareness of food allergies and anaphylaxis along with promoting education and research. A portion of the FAAN's Web site is designed for kids and teens: *www.fankids.org/*

National Heart, Lung, and Blood Institute (NHLBI)

NHLBI Information Center, National Institutes of Health,
  PO Box 30105, Bethesda, MD 20824-0105

1-301-251-1222

www.nhlbi.nih.gov/

The NHLBI is the primary NIH organization responsible for research on asthma and is the sponsor of the NAEPP (National Asthma Education and Prevention Program) discussed in the text. You can:

Read the *Expert Panel Report* at

www.nhlbi.nih.gov/guidelines/asthma/asthgdln.htm

Calculate your BMI (body mass index) at

www.nhlbisupport.com/bmi

Learn about severe asthma research at

http://patientrecruitment.nhlbi.nih.gov/CC/asthma-research.htm

More Useful Web Resources

All Allergy

A portal with many links to a variety of organizations involved in all phases of allergy and asthma. There are subjects suitable for younger children and teenagers.

www.allallergy.net

Centers for Disease Control and Prevention (CDC)

The Centers for Disease Control and Prevention has a very informative site on asthma. It includes reliable, up-to-date, comprehensive information on all aspects of asthma, for all age groups.

www.cdc.gov/asthma/

The CDC site includes a special part for schools and childcare providers.

www.cdc.gov/asthma/schools.html

The CDC also maintains a Web site with the most up-to-date information on influenza and influenza vaccination.

www.cdc.gov/flu

ChestNet

The American College of Chest Physicians' (ACCP) Web site, ChestNet, has educational materials on many aspects of asthma, including on how to use inhalers correctly.

Read and download the Patient Education Guide, *Controlling your Asthma* that includes explanations (with pictures) of how to use your inhaler.

www.chestnet.org/downloads/patients/guides/controllingYourAsthma_eng.pdf

The ACCP's educational guide on lung health (with a focus on both asthma and tobacco prevention) for students in 3rd through 6th grades, *Educational Guide on Lung Health for Elementary School Students* is addressed to teachers, school nurses, and parents and it is presented in both English and Spanish.

www.chestfoundation.org/foundation/tobacco/lungHealth.php

www.chestnet.org/downloads/patients/guides/lunghealth_eng/healthy_lungs_guide.pdf

Clinical Trials.gov

Lists ongoing investigational studies of asthma and provides information on how to participate.

www.clinicaltrials.gov/ct/gui/cation/FindCondition?ui=D001249&recruiting=true

Consortium on Asthma Camps

A helpful site for campers and their parents.

www.asthmacamps.org/asthmacamps/index.asp?topic=consortiumhome

The Consortium on Children's Asthma Camps maintains a listing of asthma camps at: *www.asthmacamps.org/asthmacamps/findacamp/usmap.asp?topic= parentsandcampers*

www.asthmacamps.org/asthmacamps/

Environmental Protection Agency (EPA)

The Environmental Protection Agency has a bilingual and user-friendly Web site on asthma with special attention to indoor and outdoor air quality. The EPA site also has a section called Managing Asthma in the School Environment.

www.epa.gov/asthma/about.html

www.epa.gov/iaq/schools/managingasthma.html

Global Initiative for Asthma (GINA)

GINA was launched in 1993 in collaboration with the National Institutes of Health (NIH) and the World Health Organization (WHO). GINA works with asthma experts worldwide to increase understanding of asthma and to improve the lives of people with asthma.

www.ginasthma.org

Hospital Web sites include the Mayo Clinic's Foundation for Medical Education and Research and the National Jewish Medical and Research Center.

www.mayoclinic.com

www.nationaljewish.org

MedlinePlus

Offers links to reliable health information on asthma from the U.S. National Library of Medicine. The up-to-date information is organized in categories such as Latest News, Disease Management, and Women, to name a few.

www.nlm.nih.gov/medlineplus/asthma.html

Also, *www.nlm.nih.gov/medlineplus/asthmainchildren.html* gives the latest information on asthma in children and young people.

National Association of School Nurses

This site contains teaching information on asthma for school staff.

1-207-833-2117

www.nasn.org

National Center for Complementary and Alternative Medicine (NCCAM)
NCCAM maintains a Web site a site under the auspices of the National Institutes
of Health (NIH). Complementary and alternative medicine is an area of great
interest and much confusion; if you are interested in ongoing complementary
and alternative medicine research in asthma, this is a good place to start.
www.nccam.nih.gov

National Jewish Health
1400 Jackson Street, Denver, CO 80206
1-303-388-4461
www.asthma.nationaljewish.org
www.nationaljewish.org/healthinfo/index.aspx
National Jewish Health's first hospital opened its doors in 1899 to treat patients
with tuberculosis and has since grown into a world-renowned respiratory hospital. Its Lung line (1-800-222-LUNG) allows you to speak to a nurse and
request that printed information and pamphlets on asthma and allergy be
mailed to you.

Peak Performance USA (PPUSA)
PPUSA is a national awareness and school asthma management program sponsored by the American Association for Respiratory Care (AARC) whose goal
is to teach students to manage their illness and lead healthier, more active
lives. The site contains information on how schools can put an asthma management program in place and provides a wealth of information on asthma.
www.peakperformanceusa.info

Pharmaceutical company–sponsored Web sites are funded by companies that
sell asthma and allergy medicines.
Examples are:
www.freebreather.com—sponsored by Schering
www.gsk.com/yourhealth/asthma.htm—sponsored by GlaxoSmithKline
www.rethinkasthmacontrol.com—sponsored by AstraZeneca

U.S. Food and Drug Administration
The FDA is a branch of the U.S. Department of Health and Human Services
and regulates several products including drugs, medical devices, and biologics.
It is a good source of information on asthma treatments.
www.fda.gov
www.fda.gov/Drugs/ResourcesForYou/Consumers/QuestionsAnswers/ucm077808.htm
reviews the latest on CFC-free HFA albuterol inhalers for asthma.

A key component of the NAEPP's asthma treatment guidelines is the classification of asthma into four separate categories based on asthma symptoms, pulmonary function test (FEV₁) values, and disease severity. An individual with asthma will fall into one of four groups at the time of the initial assessment of their asthma severity: intermittent asthma, mild persistent asthma, moderate persistent asthma, or severe persistent asthma. Interestingly, that person's classification may change over time depending on how effectively the disease and its symptoms become controlled. Patients at any level of severity can also experience exacerbations, which can be mild, moderate, or severe in intensity. The accurate classification of a person's asthma severity at the time of diagnosis and ongoing follow-up evaluations of disease control as treatment proceeds is part of the NAEPP's effort to ensure better care for persons of all ages with asthma. The NAEPP recommends specific medications and interventions for each level of asthma severity.

Table A-1   The NAEPP Classification of Intermittent Asthma

Intermittent asthma: classification in children 0–4 years of age

Symptoms

- Daytime symptoms: ≤2 days in a week
- Nighttime symptoms: none
- Need for short-acting β_2 bronchodilator for symptoms control: ≤2 days/week
- Interference with normal activities and daily routine: none

Exacerbations

- From 0 to 1 per year

Treatment (Step 1) Step 1 treatment is indicated for the initial treatment of intermittent asthma.

- All children with asthma should be prescribed inhaled quick-relief, short-acting bronchodilator therapy to be used on an as-needed basis. A short-acting, inhaled β_2 agonist is the recommended quick-relief agent.
- No daily medication needed.

Any child with intermittent asthma can experience exacerbations. The exacerbations may be mild, moderate, or even severe, but they are usually brief, lasting from hours to a few days. Treatment of any exacerbation is mandatory and will require additional medication. A short course of oral corticosteroids may be needed. Between exacerbations, a child who has intermittent asthma is asymptomatic. There can be long periods of normal lung function without any symptoms between exacerbations.

(continued)

Table A-1   The NAEPP Classification of Intermittent Asthma (*Continued*)

Intermittent asthma: classification in children 5–11 years of age

Symptoms

- Daytime symptoms: ≤ 2 days in a week
- Nighttime symptoms: ≤ 2 times a month
- Need for short-acting β_2 bronchodilator for symptoms control: ≤ 2 days/week
- Interference with normal activities and daily routine: none

Lung function tests

- Normal forced expiratory volume (FEV_1) between exacerbations
- Forced expiratory volume (FEV_1) >80% of predicted
- FEV_1/FVC ratio >85% of predicted

Exacerbations

- Fewer than 2 per year

Treatment (Step 1) Step 1 treatment is indicated for the initial treatment of intermittent asthma.

- All children with asthma should be prescribed inhaled, quick-relief, short-acting bronchodilator therapy to be used on an as-needed basis. A short-acting inhaled β_2 agonist is the recommended quick-relief agent.
- No daily medication needed.

Any child with intermittent asthma can experience exacerbations. The exacerbations may be mild, moderate, or even severe, but they are usually brief, lasting from hours to a few days. Treatment of any exacerbation is mandatory and will require additional medication. A short course of oral corticosteroids may be needed. Between exacerbations, measurement of lung function is normal, and a child who has intermittent asthma is asymptomatic. There can be long periods of normal lung function without any symptoms between exacerbations.

Intermittent asthma: classification in people 12 years and older (including all adults)

Symptoms

- Daytime symptoms: ≤ 2 days in a week
- Nighttime symptoms: ≤ 2 times a month
- Need for short-acting β_2 bronchodilator for symptoms control: ≤ 2 days/week
- Interference with normal activities and daily routine: none

Lung function tests

- Normal forced expiratory volume (FEV_1) between exacerbations
- Forced expiratory volume (FEV_1) >80% of predicted
- FEV_1/FVC ratio normal

Exacerbations

- Fewer than 2 per year

Treatment (Step 1) Step 1 treatment is indicated for the initial treatment of intermittent asthma.

- All youths and adults with asthma should be prescribed inhaled, quick-relief, short-acting bronchodilator therapy to be used on an as-needed basis. A short-acting, inhaled β_2 agonist is the recommended quick-relief agent.
- No daily medication needed.

Any youth or adult with intermittent asthma can experience exacerbations. The exacerbations may be mild, moderate, or even severe, but they are usually brief, lasting from hours to a few days. Treatment of any exacerbation is mandatory and will require additional medication. A short course of oral corticosteroids may be needed. Between exacerbations, measurement of lung function is normal, and the youth who has mild, intermittent asthma is asymptomatic. There can be long periods of normal lung function without any symptoms between exacerbations.

Table A-2   The NAEPP Classification of Mild Persistent Asthma

Mild persistent asthma: classification in children 0–4 years of age

Symptoms

- Daytime symptoms: >2 days in a week, but not daily
- Nighttime symptoms: 1 to 2 times a month
- Need for short-acting β_2 bronchodilator for symptoms control >2 days in a week, but not daily
- Interference with normal activities and daily routine: + minor limitation

Exacerbations

- 2 or more in 6 months that required taking oral steroids, or 4 or more wheezing episodes per year lasting more than 24 hours

Treatment (Step 2) Step 2 treatment is indicated for the initial treatment of mild persistent asthma.

- All children with asthma should be prescribed inhaled, quick-relief bronchodilator therapy to be used on an as-needed basis. A short-acting, inhaled β_2 agonist is the recommended quick-relief agent.
- Daily medication is required for treatment of mild persistent asthma. In most cases, low-dose inhaled anti-inflammatory medication is preferred. Montelukast or cromolyn can be alternatives.
- Consultation with an asthma specialist may be considered.

Any child with mild persistent asthma can experience exacerbations. The exacerbations may be mild, moderate, or even severe. Treatment of any exacerbation is mandatory and will require additional medication. A course of oral corticosteroids may be needed.

(continued)

Table A-2   The NAEPP Classification of Mild Persistent Asthma (*Continued*)

Mild persistent asthma: classification in children 5–11 years of age

Symptoms

- Daytime symptoms: >2 days in a week, but not daily
- Nighttime symptoms: 3 to 4 times a month
- Need for short-acting β_2 bronchodilator for symptoms control: >2 days in a week, but not daily
- Interference with normal activities and daily routine: + minor limitation

Lung function tests

- Forced expiratory volume (FEV_1) >80% of predicted
- FEV_1/FVC ratio >80% of predicted

Exacerbations

- 2 or more per year

Treatment (Step 2) Step 2 treatment is indicated for the initial treatment of mild persistent asthma.

- All children with asthma should be prescribed inhaled, quick-relief bronchodilator therapy to be used on an as-needed basis. A short-acting, inhaled β_2 agonist is the recommended quick-relief agent.
- Daily medication is required for treatment of mild persistent asthma. In most cases, low-dose inhaled anti-inflammatory medication is preferred. Pills such as leukotriene modifiers or sustained-release theophylline tablets can be alternatives along with inhaled cromolyn or nedocromil.

Any child with mild persistent asthma can experience exacerbations. The exacerbations may be mild, moderate, or even severe. Treatment of any exacerbation is mandatory and will require additional medication. A course of oral corticosteroids may be needed.

Mild persistent asthma: classification in people 12 years and older (including all adults)

Symptoms

- Daytime symptoms: more than 2 days in a week, but not daily
- Nighttime symptoms: 3 to 4 times a month
- Need for short-acting β_2 bronchodilator for symptoms control: >2 days in a week, but not daily
- Interference with normal activities and daily routine: + minor limitation

Lung function tests

- Forced expiratory volume (FEV_1) ≥80% of predicted
- FEV_1/FVC ratio normal

Exacerbations

- 2 or more per year

Treatment (Step 2) Step 2 treatment is indicated for the initial treatment of mild persistent asthma.

- All children and adults with asthma should be prescribed inhaled, quick-relief bronchodilator therapy to be used on an as-needed basis. A short-acting, inhaled β_2 agonist is the recommended quick-relief agent.
- Daily medication is required for treatment of mild persistent asthma. In most cases, low-dose inhaled anti-inflammatory medication is preferred. Pills such as leukotriene modifiers or sustained-release theophylline tablets can be alternatives along with inhaled cromolyn or nedocromil.

Any youth or adult with mild persistent asthma can experience exacerbations. The exacerbations may be mild, moderate, or even severe. Treatment of any exacerbation is mandatory and will require additional medication. A course of oral corticosteroids may be needed.

Table A-3   The NAEPP Classification of Moderate Persistent Asthma

Moderate persistent asthma: classification in children 0–4 years of age

Symptoms

- Daytime symptoms: daily
- Nighttime symptoms: 3 to 4 times a month
- Need for short-acting β_2 bronchodilator for symptoms control: daily
- Interference with normal activities and daily routine: + some limitation

Exacerbations

- 2 or more in 6 months requiring oral steroids, or 4 or more wheezing episodes per year

Treatment (Step 3) Step 3 treatment is indicated for the initial treatment of moderate persistent asthma; an oral corticosteroid burst should also be considered.

- All children with asthma should be prescribed inhaled, quick-relief bronchodilator therapy to be used on an as-needed basis in addition to daily control medicine. A short-acting, inhaled β_2 agonist is the recommended quick-relief agent.
- Daily medication is required for treatment of moderate persistent asthma. The treating physician will prescribe a regimen based on the patient's individual asthma characteristics. Medium-dose inhaled corticosteroid anti-inflammatory medication is preferred.
- Consultation with an asthma specialist is recommended.

Any child with moderate persistent asthma can experience exacerbations. The exacerbations may be mild, moderate, or even severe. Treatment of any exacerbation is mandatory and will require additional medication. A course of oral corticosteroids may be needed.

Moderate persistent asthma: classification in children 5–11 years of age

(continued)

Table A-3   The NAEPP Classification of Moderate Persistent Asthma (*Continued*)

Symptoms

- Daytime symptoms: daily
- Nighttime symptoms: >1 night in a week, but not every night
- Need for short-acting β_2 bronchodilator for symptoms control: daily
- Interference with normal activities and daily routine: + some limitation

Lung function tests

- Forced expiratory volume (FEV_1) >60% to 80% predicted
- FEV_1/FVC ratio between 75%–80%

Exacerbations

- 2 or more per year

Treatment (Step 3) Step 3 treatment is indicated for the initial treatment of moderate persistent asthma; an oral corticosteroid burst should also be considered.

- All children with asthma should be prescribed inhaled, quick-relief bronchodilator therapy to be used on an as-needed basis in addition to daily control medicine. A short-acting, inhaled β_2 agonist is the recommended quick-relief agent.
- Daily medication is required for treatment of moderate persistent asthma. The treating physician will prescribe a regimen based on the patient's individual asthma characteristics. One recommended regimen includes a medium-dose inhaled corticosteroid or a low-dose, inhaled corticosteroid combined with a long-acting, inhaled β_2 agonist bronchodilator. Alternatives can be reviewed with the treating physician and include a low-dose, inhaled corticosteroid combined with a second oral medicine.
- Refer children with moderate, persistent asthma to a physician who is an asthma specialist.

Any child with moderate persistent asthma can experience exacerbations. The exacerbations tend to last for several days. Treatment of any exacerbation is mandatory and will require additional medication, such as oral corticosteroids.

Moderate persistent asthma: classification in people 12 years and older (including all adults)

Symptoms

- Daytime symptoms: daily
- Nighttime symptoms: >1 night a week, but not every night
- Need for short-acting β_2 bronchodilator for symptoms control: daily
- Interference with normal activities and daily routine: + some limitation

Lung function tests

- Forced expiratory volume (FEV_1) >60% to 80% predicted
- FEV_1/FVC ratio reduced by 5% or more from normal

Exacerbations

- 2 or more per year

Treatment (Step 3) Step 3 treatment is indicated for the initial treatment of moderate persistent asthma; an oral corticosteroid burst should also be considered.

- All youths and adults with asthma should be prescribed inhaled, quick-relief bronchodilator therapy to be used on an as-needed basis in addition to daily control medicine. A short-acting, inhaled β_2 agonist is the recommended quick-relief agent.

- Daily medication is required for treatment of moderate persistent asthma. The treating physician will prescribe a regimen based on the patient's individual asthma characteristics. One recommended regimen includes a medium-dose inhaled corticosteroid or a low-dose, inhaled corticosteroid combined with a long-acting, inhaled β_2 agonist bronchodilator. Alternatives can be reviewed with the treating physician and include a low-dose, inhaled corticosteroid combined with a second oral medicine.

- Consider referral of youths with moderate, persistent asthma to a physician who is an asthma specialist.

Any youth or adult with moderate persistent asthma can experience exacerbations. The exacerbations tend to last for several days. Treatment of any exacerbation is mandatory and will require additional medication such as oral corticosteroids.

Table A-4   The NAEPP Classification of Severe Persistent Asthma

Severe persistent asthma: classification in children 0–4 years of age

Symptoms

- Daytime symptoms: daily, throughout the day
- Nighttime symptoms: more than once in a week
- Need for short-acting β_2 bronchodilator for symptoms control: several times daily
- Interference with normal activities and daily routine: + very limited

Exacerbations

- 2 or more in 6 months requiring oral steroids, or 4 or more wheezing episodes per year lasting 24 hours or more

Treatment (Step 3) Step 3 treatment is indicated for the initial treatment of severe persistent asthma; an oral corticosteroid burst should also be considered.

- All children with asthma should be prescribed inhaled, quick-relief bronchodilator therapy to be used on an as-needed basis addition to daily control medicine. A short-acting, inhaled β_2 agonist is the recommended quick-relief agent.

- Daily medication is required. The treating physician will prescribe a regimen based on the patient's individual asthma characteristics. Medium-dose inhaled corticosteroid anti-inflammatory medication is preferred.

- Children with severe persistent asthma should be under the care of an asthma specialist.

Any child with severe persistent asthma can experience exacerbations. The exacerbations tend to last for several days. Treatment of any exacerbation is mandatory and will require additional medication such as oral corticosteroids.

(continued)

Table A-4   The NAEPP Classification of Severe Persistent Asthma (*Continued*)

Severe persistent asthma: classification in children 5–11 years of age

Step 4–6 treatment is indicated for severe, persistent asthma.

Symptoms

- Daytime symptoms: daily, throughout the day
- Nighttime symptoms: often nightly, 7 times a week
- Need for short-acting β_2 bronchodilator for symptoms control: several times daily
- Interference with normal activities and daily routine: + very limited

Lung function tests

- Forced expiratory volume (FEV_1) <60% of predicted
- FEV_1/FVC ratio <75% of predicted

Exacerbations

- More than 2 per year

Treatment (Step 3 or 4) Step 3 or step 4 treatment is indicated for the initial treatment of severe persistent asthma; an oral corticosteroid burst should also be considered.

- All children with asthma should be prescribed inhaled, quick-relief bronchodilator therapy to be used on an as-needed basis in addition to daily control medicine. A short-acting, inhaled β_2 agonist is the recommended quick-relief agent.
- Daily medication is required. The treating physician will prescribe a regimen based on the patient's individual asthma characteristics. One suggested regimen includes a high-dose, inhaled corticosteroid combined with a long-acting, inhaled β_2 agonist bronchodilator. Some youths will also need a daily dose of oral corticosteroid. Alternatives can be discussed with the physician. The treating physician may also suggest the addition of omalizumab (in older children) if allergy is playing a significant role in asthma.
- Children with severe persistent asthma should be under the care of an asthma specialist.

Any child with severe persistent asthma can experience exacerbations. The exacerbations tend to last for several days. Treatment of any exacerbation is mandatory and will require additional medication such as oral corticosteroids.

Severe persistent asthma: classification in people 12 years and older (including all adults)

Step 4–6 treatment is indicated for severe, persistent asthma.

Symptoms

- Daytime symptoms: throughout the day
- Nighttime symptoms: often nightly, 7 times a week
- Need for short-acting β_2 bronchodilator for symptoms control: several times daily
- Interference with normal activities and daily routine: + very limited

Lung function tests

- Forced expiratory volume (FEV_1) <60% of predicted
- FEV_1/FVC ratio reduced by more than 5% from normal

Exacerbations

- 2 or more per year

Treatment (Step 4 or 5) Step 4 or step 5 treatment is indicated for the initial treatment of severe persistent asthma; an oral corticosteroid burst should also be considered.

- All youths and adults with asthma should be prescribed inhaled, quick-relief bronchodilator therapy to be used on an as-needed basis in addition to daily control medicine. A short-acting, inhaled β_2 agonist is the recommended quick-relief agent.
- Daily medication is required. The treating physician will prescribe a regimen based on the patient's individual asthma characteristics. One suggested regimen includes a high-dose inhaled corticosteroid combined with a long-acting, inhaled β_2 agonist bronchodilator. Some youths will also need a daily dose of oral corticosteroid. Alternatives can be discussed with the physician. The treating physician may also suggest the addition of omalizumab if allergy is playing a significant role in asthma.
- Youths and adults with severe persistent asthma should be under the care of an asthma specialist.

Any youth or adults with severe persistent asthma can experience exacerbations. The exacerbations tend to last for several days. Treatment of any exacerbation is mandatory and will require additional medication such as oral corticosteroids.

Appendix 2

Glossary

ABG: An acronym for arterial blood gas. The body's arteries carry oxygen-rich (O_2-rich) and carbon dioxide-poor (CO_2-poor) blood to our organs and tissues. An ABG tests a sample of blood taken directly from an artery. The measured values of O_2 and CO_2 in the ABG sample let a doctor know how well the lungs are functioning in getting the O_2 into the body and the CO_2 out. The ABG assesses how much O_2 and CO_2 are in the arterial system, which is a reflection of the efficiency and function of the respiratory system.

Actuation: The action that releases a dose of medication from a metered-dose inhaler (MDI).

Acute: Short-lived, brief, sudden, not drawn out. Chronic is the opposite of acute. A virus such as influenza will cause an acute illness that may last a few weeks. Asthma is an example of a non-acute or chronic condition. Although its symptoms may recede, asthma lasts indefinitely.

Agonist: A drug that exerts its actions by combining with specific sites (called receptors) in the body. Albuterol, for example, attaches to the lungs' β_2 receptors. By attaching to the β_2 receptors, albuterol exerts its bronchodilatory effects and causes narrowed bronchial passages to dilate or open up. Stimulation of the lungs' β_2 receptors leads to rapid relief of wheezing, tightness, and bronchoconstriction. Medicines such as albuterol are called β (beta) agonists since they fit the β_2 receptor and exert their effects through activation of the receptor sites.

Air trapping: A potentially reversible phenomenon that develops in the lungs of patients with poorly controlled or uncontrolled asthma. Air trapping can be detected on chest CT scans but is best assessed by pulmonary function test measurements. Air trapping reflects uneven lung emptying as certain areas of lung take longer to empty of air before they fill up again with the next breath. Any process that effectively narrows the caliber of the bronchial passageways can lead to air trapping. Examples of those processes include bronchoconstriction as well as accumulation of mucus in the bronchial tubes.

Albuterol: The generic name for a β_2 agonist medication that acts on the respiratory passages to cause bronchodilatation. It is classified as a quick-relief, fast-acting medicine and is extensively prescribed in the treatment of bronchial asthma. Albuterol should be taken to relieve earliest symptoms of chest discomfort, cough, wheeze, or sensations of tightness due to asthma. It is usually delivered either by a nebulizer or by a metered-dose inhaler, but an oral form also exists.

Allergen: An agent that is able to produce an abnormal (allergic) response in a susceptible individual when that person becomes exposed to the agent. An allergen is usually a protein, and it can be of various origins. Foods, drugs, and chemicals, for example, can act as allergens in certain persons. So can substances of plant or animal origin. Examples of allergens include peanut, penicillin, ragweed, and cat dander. The key concept is that allergens are not universal. In other words, an allergen leads to an allergic response only in susceptible persons. Allergens are also asthma triggers for persons with asthma and allergy.

Allergenic: Capable of causing an abnormal (allergic) response in a susceptible (allergic) individual. Some substances are considered to be more allergenic than others, meaning that those substances are known to more frequently lead to allergy symptoms in general. Pediatricians, for example, know which foods are more inherently allergenic that others, and so generally advise introducing them later in a child's diet, and only very gradually at first. Tree nuts, fish, and eggs are more allergenic in very young children than other foods such as rice, banana, beef, or green beans, and are added to the menu as a child grows older.

Allergic rhinitis: A manifestation of allergy expressed as nasal symptoms with itching, runny nose, and congestion. When due to seasonal airborne allergens, allergic rhinitis is sometimes referred to as "hay fever" or "rose fever." *See also* rhinitis.

Allergist: A physician specialized in the diagnosis and treatment of persons with allergies. Many practicing allergists in the United States have special training first in pediatrics, followed by additional qualifications in allergy. Although they treat patients in all age groups, pediatric allergists have a particular interest and expertise in allergies in children. Since many (if not most) allergies are first diagnosed in childhood, it makes sense to have the extra dual medical background.

Allergy: The body's physical response to specific external substances known as allergens. Allergens are harmless to non-allergic persons. Allergy involves the body's production of a specific antibody in direct response to a specific allergen. The result of the allergy–antibody interaction includes inflammatory and immune changes.

Those changes, in turn, lead to symptoms that may affect the eyes (allergic conjunctivitis), nose (allergic rhinitis), sinuses (allergic sinusitis), skin (eczema, hives, atopic dermatitis), and lungs (asthma triggers or allergic asthma).

Allergy testing: Methods of diagnosing allergies. Allergy tests can be obtained by two general methods: either *directly* on the patient or *indirectly* through a blood sample (RAST or ImmunoCAP) drawn from a vein. Direct tests include two different techniques: the prick (also called the prick-puncture) test and the intradermal test. Direct tests are the most sensitive way of determining whether a person has become sensitized to a specific allergen (such as peanut, cat, or ragweed). Direct tests are performed most often on either the forearm (for prick-puncture testing) or the upper arm (for intradermal testing).

Allopath: A physician graduate of an allopathic medical school. The majority of medical schools in the United States are allopathic and confer the MD degree. The original meaning of allopath is that of a physician trained in (or who practices) allopathy. Allopathy historically involved treating diseases with remedies that produced effects different from those produced by the disease itself.

Alveolar-capillary membrane: The alveolar-capillary membrane is the interface between the alveolar surface and the blood circulation. It permits rapid, nearly instantaneous exchange of oxygen, carbon dioxide, and other gases between the air-filled alveoli and the body's blood circulation running through the capillary blood vessels. The alveolar-capillary membrane is destroyed in diseases such as emphysema but is unaffected by well-controlled asthma.

Alveolus (plural: alveoli): An alveolus is a lung's air sac. Oxygen is exchanged for carbon dioxide in the lung alveoli. A dense network of capillary vessels surrounds each alveolus. The close arrangement allows for very rapid exchange (or diffusion) of oxygen from alveolus to capillary, and of carbon dioxide from capillary to alveolus. A healthy adult human lung contains approximately 300 million alveoli. The average diameter of a human alveolus is one quarter of a millimeter. The total alveolar surface available for gas exchange in a healthy adult approximates 100 meters^2, which is about the size of a tennis court.

Anabolic steroids: Compounds normally produced by the healthy body that have the capacity to increase muscle mass, among other effects. Athletes have sometimes inappropriately taken anabolic steroids as supplements in order to build strength, endurance, and muscle mass. Anabolic steroids are unrelated to the corticosteroids used in asthma treatment but are sometimes confused with such medications because of the common use of steroids to refer to both types of compounds.

Anaphylaxis: The most severe form of an allergic reaction or response. If untreated, anaphylaxis can be fatal. The term *anaphylactic shock* is sometimes used to describe the most dramatic and serious form of anaphylaxis.

Anaphylaxis usually involves several organ systems, including the cardiovascular system, the skin, the respiratory system, and the gastrointestinal tract. Symptoms include a dangerous drop in blood pressure (hypotension), hives (urticaria) with itching and rash, respiratory distress and wheezing, throat tightness, nausea, vomiting, and abdominal pain. Immediate emergency treatment is imperative. Persons at risk for the development of anaphylaxis, such as persons known to have had a prior significant allergic reaction to peanut or bee stings for example, should always have injectable epinephrine on hand. If an anaphylactic reaction were to occur, prompt injection of epinephrine under the skin is life saving.

Antagonist: Something that opposes or resists the action of another. In medicine, an antagonist is a compound that prevents the effects or actions of a different compound; e.g., antihistamine antagonizes the effects of histamine.

Antibody: A protein molecule produced in blood or in tissues in direct response to a foreign substance or antigen. A specific antigen leads to the production of a corresponding specific antibody. The production of antibody can be beneficial or deleterious, depending on the circumstances. Antibody made in response to an infectious agent—measles, for example—will protect against a second measles infection or a recurrence. Antibody made in response to common environmental agents such as pollens, grasses, mold, and animal dander may lead to the development of allergy. Only susceptible persons (allergic or atopic individuals) will actually produce antibody against common allergens. The presence of antibody in response to a particular antigen is referred to as "sensitization" to that particular antigen. When such a person goes on to develop an allergy to that allergen, the antibody is usually of the IgE class.

Antihistamine: The class of medicines that counteract the effects of histamine by blocking histamine receptors on cells, which, in turn, prevents symptoms such as sneezing, runny nose, or watering eyes. Antihistamines are most effective when taken before symptoms develop.

Arterial: Related to one or more arteries. The body's arterial circulation leaves the heart via a major artery named the aorta. The arterial circulation provides the body, its organs, and tissues with (O_2) oxygen-rich blood. The arterial system complements the venous circulation.

Aspirin: Originally, Bayer's trademark for acetylsalicylic acid, a medicine with anti-inflammatory properties. Rather than refer to the Bayer brand, aspirin now refers to any preparation of acetylsalicylic acid. Aspirin has analgesic and antipyretic properties; it is prescribed to relieve pain and fever. Because of its anti-inflammatory actions, it is also used in the treatment of rheumatoid arthritis and juvenile rheumatoid arthritis, as well as in the treatment of many forms of heart disease. Its use is contraindicated in any person with aspirin-sensitive asthma.

Asthma: A chronic respiratory condition characterized by breathing symptoms of varying intensity and frequency. Originally derived from the phrase *difficult breathing*. Asthma has a strong genetic (inherited) basis, although environmental influences play an important role as well. Asthma frequently goes hand in hand with allergy, especially in younger age groups.

Asthmagenic: A situation or substance that has the potential to trigger or bring on asthma symptoms, e.g., exercise, exposure to cold air, or response to an allergen.

Asymptomatic: Without any manifestations or symptoms of disease or illness. The major goal of asthma treatment is to achieve an asymptomatic state so that the person with asthma experiences no symptoms whatsoever and is able to lead a full and productive life.

Atopy: An inherited predisposition to the development of allergic conditions such as hay fever, eczema, allergic rhinitis, and even certain forms of asthma. A person with evidence of atopy is said to be atopic.

Auscultation: The process of listening to the chest through a stethoscope. Auscultation is performed by the examiner placing a stethoscope on the skin overlying the lungs and having the patient breathe in and out.

Baseline hyperreactivity: Baseline hyperreactivity (BHR) is a key characteristic of asthma. BHR refers to asthmatic lungs' innate tendency to react to certain stimuli with an inflammatory response, that in turn leads to typical asthma symptoms, including breathlessness, chest tightness, breathing discomfort, cough, and wheezing. Asthma and a state of increased baseline hyperreactivity go hand in hand. BHR can be conceptualized as the asthmatic lungs' greater sensitivity to inhaled substances that would produce no effect in a healthy person without asthma. A person with asthma, for example, might start to experience uncomfortable breathing when entering a room where people are smoking cigarettes, or when running outdoors to catch a bus in subzero temperatures. Their friends, who are accompanying them to the party, or sprinting alongside to catch the bus, have no respiratory discomfort in the same situations. Physicians can assess BHR, in part, with a special pulmonary function test—the methacholine challenge (or bronchoprovocation) test. Scientists and physicians hope that future research into BHR might yield treatments that would modify or lessen the increased BHR that is characteristic of asthma.

Body mass index (BMI): A mathematical formula based on height and weight. BMI is a tool used in population studies of obesity because of its ease of measurement. The BMI in most individuals correlates to measures of body fat. To calculate your BMI, you can use either metric or conventional American units. You need to know your weight measured in kilograms or in pounds, and your height measured in meters or inches. Then use one of the formulae below:

$$**BMI = \text{weight in kilograms} \div (\text{height in meters} \times \text{height in meters})$$

**BMI = weight in pounds ÷ (height in inches × height in inches) × 703.

Obesity can be defined based on a person's BMI. An adult with a BMI of between 25 and 30 is considered overweight, and an adult with a BMI of 30 or greater meets criteria for a diagnosis of obesity. Note that BMI is used differently in children and adolescents. The interpretation of BMI values in children and adolescents requires an adjustment for age.

Bronchial passages: The breathing tubes of the lungs.

Bronchial thermoplasty: An emerging treatment option for refractory, steroid-resistant asthma. It is a minimally invasive outpatient procedure performed through a bronchoscope and targets airway smooth muscle with radio-frequency generated heat.

Bronchiectasis: A lung disease that causes abnormal, permanent dilatation of the small bronchiolar air tubes and passages that lead to the lung alveoli. Bronchiectasis causes a wide spectrum of disease. In its mildest form, bronchiectasis can be inapparent, asymptomatic, and silent. When extensive, bronchiectasis can lead to recurrent lung infection, along with symptoms of breathlessness, cough, mucus production, and wheezing.

Bronchiole: The fine, tapered, thin-walled breathing passages that branch and extend from the bronchus, and end in the alveolar air sacs.

Bronchiolitis: An inflammation of the tiniest bronchial tubes. Bronchiolitis can be secondary to an infection (infectious bronchiolitis), or from a noninfectious cause such as cigarette smoking (smoker's bronchiolitis).

Bronchitis: An inflammation of the lining of the larger bronchial tubes. Bronchitis can be acute, as from infection, or chronic, as in the case of tobacco abuse. Chronic obstructive bronchitis is the correct American term for the cigarette-related type of COPD that demonstrates obstructive dysfunction on PFTs and that causes symptoms of cough, mucus production, breathlessness, and episodes of wheezing.

Bronchoconstriction: An abnormal narrowing of the air passages. Bronchoconstriction is a prominent characteristic of asthma and is due to an increased inflammatory response in the lung.

Bronchodilatation: A widening or opening up of the lung air passages; the reverse of bronchoconstriction. Bronchodilator medicines improve breathing and relieve asthma symptoms by opening and restoring the caliber of abnormally narrowed (constricted) bronchi.

Bronchoprovocation test: A specialized pulmonary function test that correlates with baseline hyperreactivity (BHR) and that can be helpful in the diagnostic evaluation of suspected asthma. Both methacholine challenge testing and cold-air exercise challenge are examples of bronchoprovocation tests.

Bronchoscopy: A procedure that allows a lung specialist to visually inspect the lungs' breathing passages (bronchi) and to obtain specimens or biopsies of any abnormalities. Bronchoscopy can also be used for therapeutic purposes, to remove mucus accumulation or inhaled foreign bodies, or to place stents in the airways in the case of abnormal narrowing.

Bronchospasm: Abnormal contraction of the bronchial smooth muscles. *See also* bronchoconstriction.

Bronchus (plural bronchi): A breathing passage or tube. The trachea splits at the level of the carina into the right and left mainstem bronchi. The right mainstem bronchus leads air to and from the entire right lung. The left mainstem bronchus leads air to and from the entire left lung. The mainstem bronchi further subdivide into bronchial tubes that lead to the subdivisions of each lung. Those bronchial tubes eventually branch out into smaller and narrower air passages called bronchioles before ending in alveoli.

Caffeine: A naturally occurring compound found in coffee and tea and added to other beverages such as soda or energy drinks. It is also added to some medications, such as those used for treatment of pain or headache. Caffeine has several effects in the body. It is a weak lung bronchodilator. It is a central nervous system stimulant, and it increases mental alertness and wakefulness. Caffeine acts as a mild kidney diuretic, leading to an increase in urine excretion.

Capillary: A tiny, thin-walled blood vessel. The word is derived from *capillus*, the Latin word for hair. The lungs' capillaries play a crucial role in

health as part of the alveolar-capillary membrane, absorbing O_2 into the body and getting rid of CO_2.

Carbon dioxide (CO_2): An odorless, colorless gas produced as a waste byproduct by the body's metabolism. Carbon dioxide is normally excreted by the lungs and should not be confused with carbon monoxide (symbol: CO), which is a poisonous, odorless gas that, when inhaled, can lead to carbon monoxide poisoning.

Cardiac asthma: An outdated term that refers to the symptoms produced by dysfunction of the left ventricle, the heart's main pumping chamber in a condition known as CHF, or congestive heart failure. The symptoms of cardiac asthma are reminiscent of those experienced by persons during an asthma exacerbation, but the symptoms are not due to asthma. In cardiac asthma, breathlessness, cough, and wheezing occur because of heart disease combined with a state of fluid retention, not because of a lung condition. As such, the term *cardiac asthma* is a misnomer.

Carina: The split where the lungs' trachea divides into two branches—the right mainstem bronchus and the left mainstem bronchus, which lead air to the right lung and left lung, respectively.

Chlorofluorocarbons (CFCs): Chemical propellants previously used in the manufacture of metered-dose inhalers. The manufacture and use of CFCs are now banned because of their harmful effects on Earth's protective ozone layer.

Chromosome: Cellular microscopic structures that contain groupings of DNA. Chromosomes carry genetic information, or genes, in their DNA. All human cells (except for a female's mature ova and a male's sperm cells) contain in their center, or nucleus, a total of 46 chromosomes, divided in 23 pairs. An individual's 46 chromosomes constitute their genome. Half of the chromosomes are inherited from the father (via the sperm cell's 23 chromosomes), and half from the mother (via the mature ovum's 23 chromosomes).

Chronic: Longstanding, lingering, or expected to last indefinitely; as opposed to acute. Asthma and hypertension are considered to be chronic illnesses, for example. Although both respond very well to treatment and can be readily brought under control, they still last indefinitely from a medical perspective.

Chronic obstructive bronchitis: Chronic obstructive bronchitis is the technically correct medical term for the cigarette-related type of COPD that demonstrates obstructive dysfunction on PFTs and that causes symptoms of cough, mucus production, breathlessness, and episodes of wheezing.

Constriction: Narrowing, the opposite of dilatation. *See also* bronchoconstriction.

COPD: An acronym for chronic obstructive pulmonary disease. COPD refers to several different lung diseases that share similar symptoms and that demonstrate a similar pattern of dysfunction on the spirometry part of PFTs. The COPD group of lung conditions includes the cigarette-related lung diseases, emphysema, and chronic obstructive bronchitis. Consequently, many persons will use the term COPD to refer to emphysema, chronic obstructive bronchitis, or both. Some even employ the term as a kind of shorthand for tobacco-related lung disease.

Corticosteroids: Corticosteroids are hormones that are normally produced in very small quantities in health by the body's adrenal glands. Corticosteroids play a role in the regulation of blood pressure, as well as in the body's salt and water balance. Corticosteroids have been synthesized in the laboratory. They are useful medicines when prescribed in the treatment of inflammatory conditions. Corticosteroids in inhaled form are a key medication used in the treatment of asthma in all age groups.

CT (computerized tomography) scan: A three-dimensional imaging technique that provides very precise anatomic detail using X-ray technology. Images of the sinuses and lungs produced by CT scanning provide physicians with accurate information about how those structures look.

Cyanosis: An abnormal physical examination finding that correlates with abnormally low levels of blood oxygen. Cyanosis is a bluish discoloration best detected in the nail beds (under the fingernails) and around the lips.

Cystic fibrosis: A congenital metabolic disorder that primarily involves the lungs and the gastrointestinal system.

Children with cystic fibrosis produce thick mucus that causes obstruction in the pancreas, liver, intestines, and lungs. Early diagnosis and treatment are critical factors for insuring the long-term survival of children with this condition.

Desensitization: Reduction or elimination of an allergic sensitivity or reaction to a specific allergen. Immunotherapy (allergy shots) is generally used to achieve desensitization in patients with allergies.

Differential diagnosis: The process of considering different conditions or diseases that could be responsible for a patient's symptoms. After reviewing the patient's history, findings of the physical examination, and laboratory and test data, a physician will generate a list of differential diagnoses. Each diagnosis on the list is a possibility, and some are more likely than others.

Diffusion: The process in which gases and liquids intermingle until a state of balance or equilibrium is obtained. During respiration, O_2 (a gas) in the alveolus diffuses into capillary blood (a liquid) in the lung, while CO_2 (another gas) diffuses out of the capillary blood into the alveolus. Diffusion of O_2 and of CO_2 occurs extremely rapidly across the alveolar-capillary membrane in healthy lungs. Several disease states can interfere with the diffusing capacity of the lung. Emphysema, for example, destroys normal lung. As diffusion becomes more and more impaired, emphysematous lungs can no longer supply enough O_2 for the body's needs. Supplemental (extra) oxygen is sometimes required in the treatment of advanced emphysema and is administered continuously via tubing and nasal prongs. Pulmonary function testing (PFT) includes an assessment of the lung's diffusion capacity in a test called, appropriately, diffusion. Although diffusion can be impaired during a significant exacerbation of asthma, diffusion measured on PFTs is generally within normal or predicted values in asthma.

Dilatation: An opening or widening; the opposite of constriction. *See also* bronchodilatation.

Dry-powder inhaler (DPI): A newer method of delivering medication directly to the lungs and respiratory passages. DPIs are supplanting traditional MDIs partly because of their ease of use, convenience, and good patient acceptance. They are breath activated and do not contain any propellant, so their manufacture does not use any ozone-depleting chlorofluorocarbons (CFCs). Several different classes of respiratory medicines are available in DPI form, including inhaled corticosteroids, long-acting β_2 agonists, and anticholinergic bronchodilators.

Dust mites: Common household allergens. They are microscopic living organisms found indoors in tempered climates, especially in mattresses, bedding, and upholstered furniture. Dust mites live off scales of human skin. Although they are a common cause of allergy and consequently of asthma exacerbation, their numbers can be greatly reduced in the home (and perhaps nearly eliminated) by straightforward control measures. Such measures might include adjustment of the home's humidity level, encasement of all bedding in special covers, laundering bedding in hot water on a regular basis, and eliminating stuffed animals along with certain types of furniture and draperies.

Dyspnea: An abnormal awareness of breathing; a kind of breathlessness. The act of breathing should be automatic and comfortable. Dyspnea is a classic symptom of asthma and should lessen once effective treatment begins.

Eczema: An allergic skin condition also known as atopic dermatitis. In babies, eczema often involves the cheeks and diaper area, whereas in older children a distribution behind the elbow creases and the area behind the knees is classic. Eczema can be very itchy and drying.

Effector cells: Specialized white blood cells (such as macrophages, T cells, B cells, and activated mast cells) that interact and release mediators that create the typical symptoms of an allergic response.

Emphysema: One of the COPD group of lung diseases. Cigarette smoking is a significant risk factor for the development of emphysema.

Endogenous steroids: Steroids normally produced in health by the body's adrenal glands. *See also* corticosteroids.

Endotracheal intubation: The procedure in which a specialized breathing tube is placed into the trachea through the mouth or the nasal passages to allow airway support and the administration of extra oxygen. Endotracheal intubation can be life saving in cases of respiratory failure. It is also performed for major surgery, typically in the operating room when a person is to receive general anesthesia.

Environmental control: One of the three components of a comprehensive management and treatment program for children with asthma. Specifically, the term refers to the avoidance or elimination from the home, school, or work environment of those substances, allergens, or irritants that are responsible for a patient's symptoms. Common targets of environmental control include dust mites, household pets, and the use of wood-burning fireplaces.

Eosinophilic pneumonia: A rare type of lung disease characterized by breathlessness and elevated eosinophil counts like asthma, but with abnormal X-ray studies, unlike asthma.

Eosinophils: White blood cells involved in combating infection by parasites as well as playing a role in allergy and asthma.

Epidemic: An outbreak of a disease that spreads abnormally quickly and extensively. If an epidemic becomes even more widespread, across continents, it is termed a *pandemic*.

Epidemiologic: Based on the study of populations or of large groups of people.

Epinephrine: A naturally occurring hormone produced by the human adrenal glands. A synthetic form (adrenaline) is used to treat severe allergic reactions (anaphylaxis) and life-threatening asthma.

Estrogens: A group of female hormones synthesized chiefly by the ovaries. Estrogens stimulate the development and maintenance of the female secondary sexual characteristics.

Exacerbation: A flare of disease activity or of disease symptoms. An exacerbation of asthma can be caused by a viral infection, for example, and would lead to increased symptoms of cough, mucus, chest tightness, and wheezing.

Exhalation: The action of breathing air out of your lungs, also called expiration. The respiratory cycle has two parts—inspiration and expiration.

Expiratory: Breathing out.

Family practitioner: A type of physician specialized in the treatment of persons of all ages. May be qualified to perform minor surgical procedures, set fractures, and deliver babies in addition to providing medical care and prescribing medicines.

FEV_1: Forced expiratory volume in 1 second, which is a subtest of the spirometry portion of the pulmonary function tests. Both the FEV_1 and a second measurement, the FEV_1/FVC ratio, are used to diagnose asthma. Measurement of the FEV_1 is used to assess asthma control and to follow response to treatment.

Flexible bronchoscopy: A type of bronchoscopy (*see also* bronchoscopy) performed with a specialized fiberoptic instrument called a flexible bronchoscope.

Fulminant: Occurring suddenly, with great intensity and severity.

Gas exchange: The process by which O_2 and CO_2 enter and leave the body, via the lungs' alveolar capillary membrane.

Gastroesophageal reflux disease (GERD): A condition that, when present, may lead to abdominal symptoms and heartburn and may also significantly worsen underlying asthma. GERD, or more simply reflux, is usually treated with a combination of dietary changes and medicine.

Gene: A unit of heredity made up of a sequence of DNA. Genes are the basic unit of inheritance. Each gene occupies a specific place (locus) on a chromosome. They are capable of duplicating themselves each time a cell divides, and genes determine a particular characteristic or trait.

Genetic: Related to a gene or a gene product. A genetic trait is an inherited characteristic that is passed from parent to child at conception.

Gestation: Another word for pregnancy, *gestation* is derived from the Latin verb *gestare*, which means to carry.

High-efficiency particulate air (HEPA) filter: Filters that meet very stringent filtration requirements. They are capable of trapping particles of very small size, including common indoor allergens, and even certain microorganisms that pose a risk to human health. HEPA filters are used in industrial settings, as well as in hospitals. In hospitals, HEPA filters are incorporated in the ventilation and exhaust systems of operating suites and isolation rooms. HEPA filters are occasionally recommended in the home

Glossary

as part of environmental control measures in treatment of allergy. Some vacuum cleaners incorporate HEPA filtration, and room-size fans that filter the room's air through the HEPA device are available.

Histamine: A naturally occurring chemical that exerts effects on muscle, blood capillaries, and stomach secretions by attaching to H_1 and H_2 receptors in the body. Most of the body's histamine is located in mast cells, which are a type of white blood cell. When histamine is released from mast cells as occurs during an allergic reaction, the released histamine attaches to the histamine receptor, and that combination causes an inflammatory response that can include bronchoconstriction in the lung (from constriction of the muscles that encircle the bronchial tubes) and wheezing, runny nose, tearing, hives, itching, and increased stomach acid production. Medicines of the antihistamine class block the attachment of histamine to the histamine receptors and effectively neutralize the inflammatory response mediated by histamine.

Hormone: A chemical substance produced in the body by specialized endocrine glands. Once synthesized, hormones circulate in the bloodstream and regulate different body functions. Insulin is a hormone, for example. It is produced in the pancreas gland and enters the blood circulation where it exerts profound effects on glucose (sugar) and carbohydrate metabolism.

Hydrofluoroalkanes (HFAs): Medically inert substances that are used as propellants in metered-dose inhalers and meet CFC-free criteria.

Hygiene hypothesis: A theory that links exposure to dirty environments and to certain infectious agents at specific times in early childhood to a decreased risk for the development of asthma. The hypothesis attempts to connect the increasing prevalence of childhood asthma with the concurrent decreased prevalence of infections in childhood.

Hyperinflation: Lung overdistention; sometimes used interchangeably with air trapping, as air trapping results in hyperinflation. Uncontrolled or poorly controlled asthma may lead to hyperinflation, which should abate and reverse with treatment.

Hyperreactivity: With respect to asthma, refers to asthmatic lungs' greater sensitivity to inhaled substances that would produce no effect in a healthy person without asthma.

Hyposensitization: One possible (favorable) outcome of allergen immunotherapy (allergy shots). It refers to a decrease, but not total elimination, of a person's ability to develop allergic symptoms to a specific allergen, which occurs as a result of an immunotherapy regimen.

Hypoxia: Decreased and abnormally low levels of oxygen in the bloodstream.

Immune system: The primary defense system of the body. The immune system is responsible for providing protection against bacteria, viruses, cancer, and any proteins that are foreign to the body. The system is composed of the thymus gland, the bone marrow, the lymph nodes (glands), the spleen, and specialized lymphoid tissue located in the intestinal tract.

Immunoglobulin: A protein produced by the body's immune system as part of an immune response to an antigen. Antigens can be infectious agents such as viruses, bacteria and parasites, or other proteins. When immunoglobulins are synthesized in response to an infection, they play a defensive and protective role. Immunoglobulins are sometimes called gamma globulins, an older term. Immunoglobulins are of five classes: IgA, IgD, IgE, IgG, and IgM.

Immunoglobulin E (IgE): A type of immunoglobulin that rises and is produced by the body in greater quantity in the setting of atopy, allergic asthma, and a typical allergic reaction.

Immunologist: A specialist in the science of immunology, which is concerned with various phenomena of immunity, sensitivity, and allergy.

Immunotherapy: One of the three main therapeutic approaches to the management of allergic disorders. Various terms have been used to describe this form of therapy, including *desensitization* (which is a misnomer), *hyposensitization*, or, most commonly, *allergy shots*. Patients are given subcutaneous injections of the specific allergens responsible for their symptoms. The purpose of the treatment is to decrease or eliminate the patient's sensitivity by stimulating the production of a protective (blocking) IgG antibody.

The average duration of successful therapy generally takes 3–5 years.

In vitro: A process carried out outside of a living organism, in a man-made environment such as a test tube or culture medium. Any test or experiment performed in a laboratory would be considered an in vitro test. Derived from the Latin word for in glass.

In vivo: Allergy tests performed by prick/puncture or intradermal technique on a patient. A term derived from the Latin meaning within a living being.

Incidence: In medicine, refers to the number of new cases of a disease at any point in time. To say, for example, that the incidence of peanut allergy increased in a certain community in the year 2010, as compared to 2009, you would need to count the number of new cases of peanut allergy in the community that were diagnosed in 2009, and compare that statistic to the number of new cases found in 2010.

Inflammation: A physiologic process that plays a very important role in asthma. Inflammation occurs as a consequence of the release of chemicals called inflammatory mediators from specialized white blood cells. The release of these chemicals, which occurs most often as the result of an allergic reaction, has the potential to cause chronic changes within the tissues of organs such as the lung. Over time, inflammation has the potential to damage organs, thereby making them less capable of performing their normal functions.

Influenza: The influenza virus and the infectious illness caused by that virus.

Influenza begins abruptly and is characterized by high fever, chills, aches, and exhaustion. The illness is preventable via vaccination.

Inspiration: The action of taking a breath of air into your lungs. The respiratory cycle has two parts: inspiration and expiration.

Inspiratory: Breathing in.

Internist: A physician specialized in the nonsurgical medical care of adults.

Larynx: The voice box. Two vocal cords allow for speech as inhaled air passes between them and sets up vibrations within the larynx located in the middle of the neck.

Leptin: A human protein identified in 1994 and named after *leptos,* the Greek word for thin. Leptin seems to play a role in the regulation of food intake, energy balance, and ultimately of weight.

Leukotriene: An inflammatory molecule. There are two families of leukotrienes. One in particular, called the cysteinyl-leukotriene, is important in asthma and allergy. Cysteinyl-leukotrienes are released in increased number during asthma exacerbations. Drugs known as leukotriene modifiers have been developed based on current knowledge of leukotrienes. The leukotriene modifiers include (1) receptor antagonists or blockers and (2) synthesis inhibitors. The first class blocks the effects of leukotrienes (blockers), while the second interferes with their formation (synthesis inhibitors). Medicines in the first category are very safe and widely used in the maintenance treatment of allergic rhinitis and asthma.

Mediators: Chemical compounds that are either preformed or actively produced by specialized white blood cells as the result of an allergic reaction. These substances are responsible for the rapid onset of symptoms such as sneeze, runny nose, tearing eyes, cough, and wheeze, and the delayed development of inflammation.

Metered-dose inhaler (MDI): Devices that allow the delivery of a precise and accurate dose of medicine to the lungs by inhalation. MDIs are reliable, portable, and very convenient. Many different types of respiratory medicines come in MDI form, including short-acting "rescue" bronchodilators, inhaled steroids, and anti-inflammatory medicines, as well as inhaled anticholinergics. Medicines in MDI form are used in the treatment of asthma and COPD. The newer MDIs use a CFC-free propellant, usually HFA.

Methacholine challenge test: A type of bronchoprovocation test. It is a specialized pulmonary function test used in the evaluation of suspected asthma, when the diagnosis is otherwise uncertain.

Morbidity: A measure of illness in a given population. The morbidity rate from a disease is defined as the proportion of people affected by that disease per year, per given unit of population.

Mortality: A measure of illness; the rate of death from a disease in a given community or population at a precise point in time. The yearly mortality rate from a disease is defined as the ratio of deaths due to that disease, to the total number of persons in that community or population.

Mucus: A mixture composed of water, salt, and proteins produced by specialized cells in the nose, sinuses, and lung passages. Mucus plays a defensive role and helps to protect from infection. Mucus can also be produced in increased quantities as a consequence of irritation of the mucus-producing glands, as often occurs transiently in asthma exacerbations, and on a more long-term basis in chronic smokers. Doctors often use the phrase *mucus hypersecretion* when extra mucus develops.

National Asthma Education and Prevention Program (NAEPP): Program that aims to improve asthma care in the United States by teaching health professionals, asthma patients, and the general public about asthma. The NAEPP was founded in 1989 under the auspices of the National Institute of Health's National Heart Lung and Blood Institute. The NEAPP's panel of experts has published several reports with guidelines for the diagnosis and management of asthma, most recently in 2007.

Nebulizer: A device that transforms a respiratory drug in liquid form into a fine mist of medicine particles that are easily inhaled into the respiratory passages. It is powered by a machine or compressor that runs off electrical current or batteries. Nebulizers are used in babies and very young children with asthma who cannot use an MDI or DPI. They are also often used in an emergency setting. Several different classes of asthma medicines are available for nebulization, including β_2 agonists and inhaled corticosteroid preparations.

Nocturnal: Taking place or occurring during the night. Asthmatic exacerbations, for example, usually include nocturnal symptoms.

Non-steroidal anti-inflammatory drugs (NSAIDs): Potent anti-inflammatory drugs, widely prescribed for the treatment of pain, fever, and conditions such as arthritis. Some NSAIDs are available over the counter; others require a physician's prescription. As a rule, NSAIDs cross-react with aspirin and are contraindicated in persons with aspirin-sensitive asthma.

Obesity: The condition of being significantly overweight. A person is obese if he or she weighs more than 30% above his or her ideal body weight for his or her given age, height, and gender. Another definition of obesity involves computation of the BMI. An overweight adult has a BMI of between 25 and 30, while an obese adult has a BMI of 30 or greater.

Obstructive dysfunction: A pattern of abnormality detected by pulmonary function testing. Several different lung conditions lead to obstructive dysfunction on spirometry, one of the PFTs. Asthma is one of the conditions that, on testing, demonstrates obstructive dysfunction. A key element of the obstructive dysfunction uniquely seen in asthma is that, by definition, the obstruction (or abnormality) is completely reversible.

Oral: By mouth. Oral medications are taken by mouth and swallowed. Once swallowed, they dissolve in the digestive tract, and become absorbed into the bloodstream. From there, they enter the organs and tissues to exert their pharmacologic effects. Oral medicines come in tablets and capsules and in chewable and liquid forms.

Osteopath: A practitioner of osteopathy, a school of medicine originally based upon the concept that the body in correct alignment becomes efficient at making its own remedies against illness. Osteopaths today are physician graduates of osteopathic medical schools. They use the designation D.O. after their names to indicate that they are doctors of osteopathy. Osteopaths are trained to use the diagnostic and therapeutic modalities of regular medicine, in addition to manipulative methods.

Osteopathy: A system of medicine that uses conventional medical remedies and is based on the theory that disturbances in the musculoskeletal system affect other body parts and lead to disease. Consequently, manipulation of the body and musculoskeletal system restores health.

Oxygen (O$_2$): An odorless, colorless gas necessary for life. The air we breathe is comprised of 21% oxygen.

Pandemic: An epidemic that has spread extensively, affecting most countries and regions of the globe. In 2009, the novel H1N1 influenza virus became so widespread that it became pandemic.

Pathologic: Abnormal finding or feature indicative of the presence of a medical condition or disease. A cough, for example, is not normal, and when present in a child is considered pathologic from a medical perspective. The science that studies the causes and the nature of diseases is the science of pathology.

Peak expiratory flow (PEF): Part of the several different measurements obtained during the spirometry portion of pulmonary function tests. Since exacerbations of asthma lead to decreasing values of PEF, home self-monitoring of PEF in asthma is part of contemporary asthma management. Measuring PEF helps guide therapy. If the PEF begins to drop, for example, a person with asthma may need to use his or her quick relief inhaler, and increase the dose of inhaled corticosteroid medication. Lightweight, home peak flow monitors are convenient and easy to use, even by children.

Pediatrician: A physician specialized in the care of children and adolescents younger than 18 years of age. Pediatricians have received training in well-baby and well-child care as well as in the diagnosis and treatment of illnesses that can affect children from birth through adolescence.

Percussion: The physical examination of the lungs includes a technique called percussion that requires gently tapping on the chest wall and listening to the quality of the sound produced. Healthy air-filled lungs are resonant to percussion. Pneumonia or a fluid collection around the lungs, on the other hand, gives rise to dullness to percussion.

Pharmacotherapy: Treatment by medication administered either by mouth, through injection, inhalation, or intravenously.

Postnatally: After birth. Human lungs continue to grow and develop postnatally, into infancy.

Prevalence: In medicine, the total number of cases of a disease diagnosed at a given point in time. Includes all cases, whether the diagnosis is new or more longstanding. To assess the prevalence of asthma in a community as of January 1, for example, you would count all persons alive on that date who were ever told by a medical professional that they had a diagnosis of asthma.

Puberty: The time during which sexual maturation occurs. Also refers to the time when reproductive organs develop to allow reproduction.

Pulmonary embolus: A clot, usually originating in the leg veins, that becomes lodged in the lung circulation. The diagnosis of pulmonary embolus can be very difficult. Pulmonary embolus leads to a variety of symptoms, which can include breathlessness and wheezing. A large or massive pulmonary embolus is a cause of sudden death.

Pulmonary function tests (PFTs): Tests that include the measurement of lung volumes, spirometry, diffusion, and sometimes ABGs.

Pulmonary infiltrates with eosinophilia (PIE): A very rare lung disease. PIE can have symptoms that mimic those of asthma. The chest X-rays and chest CT scans are abnormal in PIE, which is one differentiating feature from asthma.

Pulmonary symptoms: Symptoms experienced by an individual and related to the lungs and to the act of breathing. Wheezing, cough, breathlessness, and mucus production are examples of pulmonary symptoms.

Pulmonologist: A physician specialist with extra training and qualifications in the diagnosis and treatment of the different lung diseases. Some pulmonologists are pediatric specialists, as well; such specialists are known as pediatric pulmonologists. Pediatric pulmonologists treat babies, children, and adolescents with lung diseases. Adult pulmonologists are internists with additional specialty training and who limit their practice to adults with respiratory conditions.

RadioAllergoSorbent Test (RAST): A trademark of Pharmacia Diagnostics that originated and developed the first RAST. It is a laboratory allergy test that detects and measures the level of IgE antibodies directed against specific antigens in a blood sample. Measuring blood RAST is one way of assessing the possible presence of an allergy. If a person is suspected of being allergic to grass, for example, his or her doctor might send a blood sample for a RAST. The doctor would request a test that would detect significant levels of IgE directed against grasses. The absence of any detectable IgE to grasses would argue against a grass allergy.

Recommended Dietary Allowance (RDA): Guidelines established by the United States National Academy of Sciences' National Research Council. The RDAs advise what nutrients males and females should eat at different ages. In 1997, The National Academy of Sciences' Institute of Medicine report introduced the concept of Dietary Reference Intakes (DRIs), which have supplanted the RDAs.

Remission: In a medical context, the subsiding of disease symptoms. A person with asthma who enters a period in which he or she experiences no asthma symptoms and is not requiring any asthma medicines has entered a period of asthma remission. The disease is still present, but it is undetectable to the patient; it has no symptoms.

Respiration: The act of breathing in (inspiration) and then out (expiration). Also refers to the process whereby the lungs exchange gases, more specifically, oxygen (O_2) and carbon dioxide (CO_2) at the level of the alveolus and the alveolar-capillary membrane.

Respiratory failure: A state or illness in which the lungs become incapable of respiration. They become unable to provide the body with needed oxygen and cannot rid the body of accumulated carbon dioxide and metabolic waste products. Respiratory failure can be acute, as after a car accident, or chronic, as in the case of emphysema. Uncontrolled asthma can result in progressive respiratory failure, a true medical emergency. Left untreated, progressive respiratory failure is fatal.

Respiratory rate: The number of breaths one takes in a minute.

Retraction: A sucking in or visible depression of the muscles in the spaces between the ribs that occurs with labored breathing.

Rhinitis: An inflammation involving the mucous membranes of the nose. Rhinitis may be allergic or nonallergic. Allergic rhinitis may be seasonal, occurring only in spring, or perennial, with symptoms that are present throughout the year. Typical examples of seasonal rhinitis include ragweed pollen allergy (hay fever) and tree or grass pollen allergy (rose fever). Perennial rhinitis symptoms may occur because of sensitivity to dust mites or a household pet. Typical symptoms include sneeze, runny nose, nasal congestion, and tearing and itching of the eyes.

Rigid bronchoscopy: A type of bronchoscopy (*see also* bronchoscopy) performed with a specialized surgical instrument called a rigid bronchoscope. Rigid bronchoscopy requires general anesthesia and is indicated under different circumstances than flexible bronchoscopy.

Sensitization: In the context of allergy, the process by which a person becomes, over time, increasingly allergic to a substance (sensitizer) through repeated exposure to that substance.

Sensitizer: A substance that causes an allergic response in an individual who has become sensitized to that specific substance by a previous exposure or multiple past exposures.

Sinus: Air-filled cavities within the human skull. Adults have several sinuses, named by location: the frontal, ethmoid, sphenoid, and maxillary sinuses. The sinuses continue to form after birth; consequently, the frontal and sphenoid sinuses are not well developed in children.

Sinusitis: An inflammation of the lining of sinuses, due most commonly to either infection (viral or bacterial sinusitis) or allergy (allergic sinusitis).

Spirometry: One of the pulmonary function tests; the most important pulmonary function test in the setting of asthma diagnosis and treatment. Spirometry measures the flow of air from the lungs as a person forcefully and fully exhales from a deep inspiration. During the performance of spirometry, a subject is first asked to take a very deep breath in, and then to blow it out, as hard and as quickly as possible. Spirometry is used to detect the presence of obstructive dysfunction. If obstructive dysfunction is present, spirometry also measures the extent of the dysfunction. An individual with well-controlled and asymptomatic asthma usually has normal values on spirometry. An exacerbation of asthma will cause the emergence of an obstructive dysfunction pattern on spirometry.

Steroid: *See* corticosteroids.

Stethoscope: A medical instrument used to amplify and listen to sounds produced by internal organs, such as the lungs, heart, or bowels during a physical examination. The process of listening through the stethoscope is called auscultation. The French physician René Laënnec (1781–1826) is credited with the invention of the stethoscope.

Symptoms: What the patient notices, experiences, and reports to his or her treating physician as abnormal or different from usual. Symptoms can relate to changes in body appearance, function, or sensation. Symptoms are always and completely subjective. Examples of symptoms include cough, pain, breathlessness, chest tightness, and fatigue.

Trachea: The scientific name for the windpipe. The uppermost portion of the trachea can be felt in the front of the neck. The trachea leads air from the back of the nose and mouth into the lungs.

Tracheomalacia: A self-correcting condition found in some newborns caused by immature development of the cartilaginous rings that provide the framework for the trachea.

Trigger: In the context of asthma, a stimulus to asthma or to allergy. For example, asthma symptoms may worsen when a person with asthma is ill with a viral respiratory infection. In that situation, the infection is considered a trigger for worsening asthma. Similarly, a person who is allergic to cats will notice itchy eyes and a runny nose triggered by entering a room with a resident cat. Part of allergy and asthma treatment involves correct identification of symptom triggers, with the goal of avoiding them as much as possible in the future.

Urticaria: The scientific name for hives, a type of skin rash. Urticaria are raised, welt-like, reddened, and intensely itchy. The most common cause of urticaria is an allergic reaction. Sometimes, urticaria are idiopathic, meaning that no cause can be identified. Urticaria are treated with anti-inflammatory medicine, antihistamines, or both.

Vaccine: A specialized preparation designed to stimulate the body's immune system to make protective antibodies directed against a specific infectious agent. Some vaccines are injected into muscle or skin; others are inhaled or swallowed. Some vaccines protect against specific viruses, such as influenza (influenza vaccine) or polio (polio vaccine); others protect against bacteria, such as Haemophilus influenzae (HiB vaccine) or Streptococcus pneumonia (pneumococcal vaccine). Some vaccines contain a live, weakened strain; others contain only a portion of the infectious agent.

Valved holding chamber (VHC): A device that facilitates the inhalation of medicine from a metered-dose inhaler (MDI). There are different brands of VHCs on the market. Ideal MDI technique requires simultaneously activating the MDI canister, releasing medicine, and inhaling as deeply as one can. Adding a VHC permits the user to first actuate the medicine and then inhale deeply as a second step. Adding a VHC makes it easier to use MDIs, improves medication delivery to the lungs, and reduces deposition of medicine on the voice box. The last fact is important as deposition of inhaler medicine in the throat and on the vocal cords not only wastes medicine, but can also lead to throat irritation and hoarseness. Some persons use the term *spacer* to describe a valved holding chamber device, although they are not synonymous.

Venous: Related to the veins. Veins are blood vessels that carry oxygen-poor and carbon dioxide-rich blood away from our organs, toward the heart and lungs, where respiration and gas exchange will take place.

Ventilator: A machine that provides respiratory support to failing lungs. Respirators can provide breaths and oxygen to patients who are critically ill. They can also be used to support breathing in a nonhospital setting. Respirator machines, or respirators, are similar, and the terms are interchangeable.

Viral: Caused by or related to a virus.

Virus: A type of infectious agent. Viruses contain a single strand of either DNA or RNA, surrounded by a protein coat. Since they only contain one strand of genetic information, viruses cannot replicate on their own, and require a host cell for replication. Different viruses have different degrees of infectivity and also infect different species. Some viruses infect plants, for example. Viruses that infect humans can cause disease. Depending on the particular virus and on the underlying health of the human, viral infections can run the gamut from mild to life threatening. Influenza virus, for example, can be fatal.

Vitamin: A substance required in minute quantities for health. Vitamins occur naturally in a wide range of foods. Vitamin deficiencies are unusual in Western society, and they reflect either a disease of the absorptive capacity of the gastrointestinal system with consequent malabsorption of nutrients or a severely restricted diet.

Vocal cord dysfunction (VCD) syndrome: A condition that can be confused with asthma. VCD syndrome's primary disturbance involves the vocal cords and their abnormal tendency to move toward each other (rather than move apart) during inspiration, or breathing in. It is important to diagnose VCD if it is present, since asthma treatments will not be effective for VCD.

Wheeze: The abnormal sound produced when air travels in and out through a narrowed breathing passage or breathing tube. The narrowing in asthma can be due to a constriction of the breathing tube or accumulated mucus, or both.

Glossary

Index

Italicized page locators noted with an *f* indicate a figure; tables are noted with a *t*.

A

AAP. *See* American Academy of Pediatrics
ABG. *See* arterial blood gases
Accolate (zafirlukast), 134*t*
AccuNeb (albuterol solution), 131*t*, 171
ACE inhibitor-induced cough, 44*t*
ACLS. *See* advanced cardiac life support
Action Plan, 62
    daily management in, 88
    key features of, 89–90
    patient education in, 87–88
    recognition in, 88
    studies of, 90–91
    types of, 89*t*
actuation, 163
acupuncture, for asthma, 194–197
adolescence, asthma in, 204–205
adults, asthma in
    NAEPP guidelines for, 101
    serious symptoms of, 117*t*
Advair (fluticasone + salmeterol), 132*t*–133*t*,
        138, 144, 151, 160–161, 189
advanced cardiac life support (ACLS),
        125
aerobic exercise, 210
Aerobid (flunisolide), 131*t*–132*t*, 138
Aerobid-M (flunisolide), 131*t*
AeroChamber Max, 164
Aerolizer, 155
aerosols, propellants in, 143
Aerospan (flunisolide), 131*t*, 133*t*
age
    asthma characteristics by, 4*t*
    H1N1 by, 226*t*
    NAEPP guidelines by, 101
    school-, 247–248, 265
    serious symptoms by, 117*t*
agonist, 48. *See also* long-acting β₂ agonists
AIA. *See* aspirin-induced asthma

air purifiers
    dust mites and, 230
    HEPA, 229–231
air trapping, 218
air travel, asthma medications during,
        216–217
airways
    hyperreactivity of, 62
    narrowing of, 38
    remodeling of, 174
    resistance of, 58*t*
    smooth muscle, 193
albuterol (Fluticasone), 129*t*, 130*t*, 131*t*,
        133*t*, 137–139, 144–149, 169, 171
    reformulated MDI, 144
    uses of, 132
albuterol solution (AccuNeb), 131*t*, 171
albuterol sulfate (ProAir, Proventil, ReliOn,
        Ventolin), 133*t*, 138, 144–145,
        146–149, 161–162
allergen, 18, 50*t*
    exposure to, 190
    indoor, 264
    -induced asthma, 109–110
allergenic, 24
allergic response, 190–191
allergic rhinitis, 49
allergies
    anti-, medicine for, 133*t*
    asthma v., 16–19
    blood testing for, 111–112
    cell mechanisms in, 27
    diagnosis of, 109
    direct testing for, 110
    environmental control of, 113
    to food, 22
    immunotherapy for, 113–114
    ISAAC, 6
    to pets, 263–265

physiological response with, 18
positive, test, 111
specific testing for, 112
symptoms of, 191
testing for, 110
treatment of, 114
allergist, 110, 114
allopath, 103
alveolar-capillary membrane, 11
alveolus, 12
Alvesco (ciclesonide), 131*t*, 133*t*
American Academy of Pediatrics (AAP),
     202
American College of Chest Physicians, 147
anabolic steroids, 176
anaphylaxis, 115–116, 190,
     216, 269
antagonist, 78
     LTRA, 134
anti-allergy medications, inhaler delivery
     of, 133*t*
antibody, 112
anticholinergics, 130*t*
antihistamine, 112
anti-inflammatory corticosteroids,
          inhaled
     daily use of, 133*t*, 159–160
     delivery of, 133*t*
appetite, 180
arformoterol (Brovana), 132*t*
arterial, 63
arterial blood gases (ABG), 124
     measurement of, 58*t*
     sampling of, 63–65
Asmanex (monometasone), 131*t*, 133*t*,
     151, 160
aspirin, 83, 83*t*
     uses of, 51
aspirin-induced asthma (AIA), 82–84
     avoiding medicines in, 83, 83*t*
     safe medicines in, 84
asthma
     acupuncture for, 194–197
     in adolescence, 204–205
     in adults, 101, 117*t*
     by age, 4*t*, 101, 117*t*, 226*t*
     allergen-induced, 109–110
     allergy v., 16–19
     aspirin-induced, 82–84
     asymptomatic, 99
     attack of, 36
     in babies, 117*t*, 251–253
     in Bronx/Harlem, 7
     caffeine and, 207–208

camps for, 260–262
cardiac, 44
causes of, 13–14
CDC rates for, 3–4
cell mechanisms in, 27
characteristics of, 31
classification types for, variants and, 74–77
complementary medicine for, 194–197
conditions mimicking, 48–49
control of, 98
COPD and, 46–47
corticosteroids for, 171–174
cough-variant, 39, 77–78, 78*t*
death and, 121–122
definition of, 2
development of, 246
diagnosis of
     in babies, 252–253
     in children, 247, 249*t*
     devices for, 63
     differential, 43–44, 44*t*, 55
     establishment of, 53, 107*t*
     tools for, 56*t*
emergency, 102, 115–116
environmental factors in, 17*f*, 18–20
EPR, 68
exacerbation of, 29*t*, 34–38, 72
exercise-induced, 78–81
factors in, 8–9
by gender, 246–247
genetics causing, 13
GERD and, 49
GINA guidelines for, 76*t*, 100*t*
herbal remedies for, 194–197
history for, 54–55
ICS in, 173*t*
incidence of, 2–5, 189
increase of, 6*t*
influenza and, 219–227
management of, key components of, 97*t*
manifestation of, 53
milk and, 249–250
mineral supplements for, 197–202
Montreal Protocol for, 141–144
myths about, 232*t*
NAEPP, 68
     classification by, 71
obesity and, 202–207
occupational, 85, 87
outgrowing, 255–256
physical examination for, 55
pregnancy and, 236, 238, 238*t*
premenstrual, 197
prevalence of, 6–7

prevention of, 20–25
  prenatal, 238–240
as psychological disease, 231–233
quiescent, 29t
risk factors for, 122t, 123
at school, 247–248, 257–259, 265
scuba diving and, 217–219
self-monitoring of, 61
severity of
  control of, 50t
  forms of, 53
sleep and, 139–140
sports and, 209–216
step down therapy, 137
studies of, 14–16
supplements for, 197–202
symptoms of, 91, 93
  assessment of, 100t
  pulmonary, 54
  serious, 117t
  from textbook, 34
treatment of, 2, 3t, 99t
  goals of, 72–73, 92–94, 98–101
  modern, 97
  new approaches to, 188–194
  optimization of, 107t
  side effects from, 179–185
trigger for, 19, 42, 96t, 97, 210, 232–233
in United States, 4t
vaccines and, 225
views of, traditional/contemporary, 28–31
vitamin supplements for, 197–202
work-related, 86
asthma action plan, 62
  daily management in, 88
  key features of, 89–90
  patient education in, 87–88
  recognition in, 88
  studies of, 90–91
  types of, 89
asthma medications, 24
  during air travel, 216–217
  breastfeeding and, 244
  case study of, 135
  in children, 259
  classification of, 128
    chart of, 130t
  dosing of, 131
  facts about, 129t
  FEV$_1$ confirmation for, 137
  guidelines of, 136
  importance of, 91
  increasing use of, 37
  indications for, 136

inhaler
  types of, 133t
  benefits of, 141
  long-term control with, 133t, 134
  method of action of, 129–130
  patents of, 138
  in pregnancy
    classification of, 241t
    safety of, 240–243
  prescription of, 128
  prolonged use of, 135
  quick-relief, 129, 131–132
    at night, 140
  trade/generic names for, 131t, 132t
asthma specialist
  for children, 253–255
  importance of, 106–109
  jobs of, 103
  as physician, 103
  during pregnancy, 236–238
  referrals to, 108
asthmagenic virus, 14
asthmatic triad, 81–82
asymptomatic asthma, 99
atopy, 87
Atrovent (ipratropium), 130t, 139
auscultation, 39
Azmacort (triamcinolone), 131t, 133t, 165
AZMATICS, 14–15

B

β$_2$ agonists, 130t
  examples of, 189
  generic/trade names of, 132t
  inhaled corticosteroids combined with, 132t
  inhaler delivery of, 133t
babies
  asthma in, 117t
    patterns of, 251–252
  diagnosis in, 252–253
  wheezing in, 251t
baseline hyperactivity, 30, 31t
beclomethasone (Qvar), 130t–131t, 133t,
    144–145
beta-blocker-induced wheeze, 44t, 50t
birth
  ETS before/after, 21–22
  lungs after, 12
Blaser, Dr. Martin, 26
blood supply, to fetus, 237
blood testing
  for allergies, 111–112
  as tool, 56t
BMI. *See* body mass index

body mass index (BMI), calculation
  of, 206–207
Boushey, Dr. Homer, 22
bowels, loose, 179
breastfeeding
  advantages of, 244
  asthma medication and, 244
  importance of, 240
breath, 10f
  CO$_2$ in, 11–12
  holding, 153
  in inhalers, 156
  machine, 169
  O$_2$ in, 11–12
breathlessness, 40, 40t
bronchial passages, 231
bronchial thermoplasty, 66, 193
bronchiectasis, 40
bronchiolitis, 23
bronchoconstriction, 28, 38
  in EIB, 80
  exacerbation of, 173
bronchodilator
  caffeine as, 208
  classification of, 128
  EPR research of, 60
  generic/trade names of, 132t
  SABA, 71, 128–131, 129t, 131t, 132,
    133t, 134
bronchoprovocation
  studies of, 58t
  test for, 62–63
bronchoscopy
  flexible, 65
  FOB, 65
  performance of, 66
  rigid, 66
  types of, 65–66
  uses of, 65
bronchospasm, 102
  EIB, 213–214
bronchus, 9
Bronx, asthma in, 7
Brovana (arformoterol), 132t
budesonide (Pulmicort), 130t,
    132t–133t, 243
budesonide-formoterol (Symbicort),
    132t–133t, 189
bursts, corticosteroids for, 130t

C

caffeine
  asthma and, 207–208
  as bronchodilator, 208

calcium, 250
cancer, risk of, 201t
capillary, 11
carbon dioxide (CO$_2$)
  in breathing, 11–12
  functions of, 64
cardiac asthma, 44
cardiac dysfunction, 44t
Caribbean, 217
CDC. See Centers for Disease Control
    and Prevention
cells
  effector, 191
  IgE and, 191
  mechanism of, 27
Centers for Disease Control and Prevention
    (CDC), asthma rates by, 3, 4t
CFCs. See chlorofluorocarbons
chest CT scan, 56t
chest X-ray, 56t, 77
children
  asthma medications in, 259
  asthma specialist for, 253–255
  camps for, 260–262
  cigarette smoking affecting,
    262–263
  classification in, 4t
  cough in, 249t
  diagnosis in, 249t
  differential diagnosis in, 247
  dyspnea in, 249t
  exercise for, 215–216, 257
  gender of, 246–247
  growth in, 250–251
  outgrowing asthma in, 255–256
  pets for, 265
  prevalence in, 101, 117t
  at school, 257–259
  school-age, wheezing in,
    247–248
  serious symptoms in, 117
  vitamins for, 250
  written plans for, 258
Chlamydia pneumoniae, 14
chlorofluorocarbons (CFCs), 142–144
chromosome, 16
chronic obstructive bronchitis, 45, 46
chronic obstructive pulmonary disorder
    (COPD), 44t, 45
  asthma and, 46–47
  medications for, 47
  treatment of, 47–48
  wheezing and, 40, 40t
ciclesonide (Alvesco), 131t, 133t

cigarette smoking, 45
  affecting children, 262–263
  during pregnancy, 239
  quitting, 238*t*, 239
Clean Air Act, 143
Clearing the Air: Asthma and Indoor Air, 21
closed-mouth technique, 156
cold air, 214
coma, 124
complementary medicine, for asthma,
    194–197
computed tomography (CT), 56
congestive heart failure, 44
Consortium of Children's Asthma
    Camps, 262
constriction, 28
COPD. *See* chronic obstructive pulmonary
    disorder
corticosteroids. *See also* inhaled corticosteroids
  anti-inflammatory inhaled
    daily use of, 133*t*, 159–160
      delivery of, 133*t*
  for asthma, 171–174
  for "bursts," 130*t*
  definition of, 78*t*
  side effects of, 179–185
cough, 35*t*
  ACE inhibitor-induced, 44*t*
  in children, 249*t*
  chronic, 42
  after jogging, 41–42
  persistent, 41–42
cough-variant asthma, 39, 77–78, 78*t*
Crolom (cromolyn), 130*t*
cromolyn (Crolom), 130*t*
CT. *See* computed tomography
cyanosis, 102
cystic fibrosis, 247

D

daily use anti-inflammatory corticosteroids,
    159–160
  inhaler delivery of, 133*t*
death
  from asthma, 121–122
  from respiratory failure, 124
  risk of, 122
desensitization, 84
diabetes, 201*t*
diagnostic testing, for asthma, 56–57
Dietary Reference Intakes (DRI), 199
differential diagnosis
  of asthma, 43–44, 55
  in children, 247

diffusion, measurement of, 58*t*
Diskus
  design of, 150
  types of, 149–151
  use of, 151–159
doses, of asthma medications, 131
DPI. *See* dry-powder inhaler
DRI. *See* Dietary Reference Intakes
dry-powder inhaler (DPI), 99
  empty, 160–163
  types of, 150
  use of, 141, 149
    correct, 151–155
dust mites, 227–231
  air purifiers and, 230
  decreasing exposure to, 229–230
  definition of, 227
  location of, 228
  survival of, 228
dyspnea, 34, 35*t*
  in children, 249*t*

E

eczema, 20
education
  in action plan, 87–88
  NAEPP, 58*t*, 59, 68, 71, 101, 188
  physical, 257
effector cells, 191
EIA. *See* exercise-induced asthma
EIB. *See* exercise-induced bronchospasm
emergency room
  case study of, 118
  going to, 115–116
  nebulizer in, 119
  PEF in, 120
  staff in, 116
  time spent in, 120
  treatment in, 119
emotional response, as trigger,
    232–233
emphysema, 45
endogenous steroids, 176
endotracheal intubation, 124
environmental factors
  in allergies, 113
  in asthma, 17*f*, 18–20
environmental tobacco smoke (ETS),
    before/after birth, 21–22
eosinophilic pneumonia, 49
eosinophils, 173
epidemic, 219
epidemiology, 14
  of hygiene hypothesis, 26

Index

EPR. *See* Expert Panel Report: Guidelines for the Diagnosis and Management of Asthma
EPR-3, 60, 68–73, 75, 87–88, 101, 107, 114, 164, 188, 258
   guidelines for, 75
   uses of, 70–72
estrogens, 172
ETS. *See* environmental tobacco smoke
exacerbated asthma, 29*t*, 34–38, 72
   key points of, 37*t*
   mild, 36
   treatment of, 36–37
exacerbation, 24
   of asthma, 29*t*, 34–38, 72
   of bronchoconstriction, 173
   symptoms of, 35, 35*t*
exercise
   aerobic, 210
   in children, 215–216, 257
   leukotriene modifiers and, 213–214
   as trigger, 42, 210
   types of, 211
   warming up before, 214
exercise-induced asthma (EIA), 78–81
exercise-induced bronchospasm (EIB), 213–214
exhalation
   definition of, 59
   measurement of, 59–60
Expert Panel Report (EPR): Guidelines for the Diagnosis and Management of Asthma, 68
   bronchodilator research by, 60
   holding chamber advice from, 164
   specialist referral in, 108
expiratory, 38

F

family practitioner, 106
fat tissue, 204
fetus
   blood supply to, 237
   nutrition for, 200
FEV. *See* pulmonary function tests
FEV_1. *See* forced expiratory volume
fiberoptic bronchoscopy (FOB), 65
fish oils, 200
Flexhaler, 154
flexible bronchoscopy, 65
Flovent (fluticasone HFA), 131*t*, 133*t*, 138, 151, 160–161
flunisolide (Aerobid, Aerobid-M, Aerospan), 130*t*–131*t*, 133*t*

Fluticasone (albuterol), 130*t*, 132*t*–133*t*, 134, 151
fluticasone + salmeterol (Advair), 132*t*–133*t*, 144, 151, 189
fluticasone HFA (Flovent), 131*t*, 133*t*, 138, 151, 160–161
FNB. *See* Food and Nutrition Board
FOB. *See* fiberoptic bronchoscopy
food, allergy to, 22
Food and Nutrition Board (FNB), 199
Foradil (formoterol DPI), 132*t*–133*t*, 151
forced expiratory volume (FEV_1), 59
   decrease of, 60
   knowing your, 70*t*
   measurement of, 60
   for medication, 137
formoterol DPI (Foradil), 130*t*, 132*t*, 144, 151
formoterol solution (Performist), 132*t*
fulminant, 221

G

GABRIEL, 27
gas exchange, 11
   measurement of, 58*t*
gastroesophageal reflux (GERD), 41, 44*t*
   asthma and, 49
   manifestations of, 52
   treatment of, 52
gender, asthma by, 246–247
gene, 16
generic names. *See also Specific drug, such as formoterol DPI*
   of β_2 agonists, 132*t*
   bronchodilator, 132*t*
   of HFA, 148*t*
   of ICS, 131*t*
   of LABA, 132*t*
   of leukotriene modifiers, 131*t*
   of medications, 131*t*–132*t*, 134*t*
   of SABA, 134*t*
   trade names v., 137–139
genetics, causing asthma, 13
GERD. *See* gastroesophageal reflux
gestation, 237
GINA. *See* Global Initiative for Asthma
GIO. *See* glucocorticoid-induced osteoporosis
Global Initiative for Asthma (GINA)
   guidelines of, 76*t*, 100*t*
   roles of, 74–75
glucocorticoid-induced osteoporosis (GIO), 181
glucose, 201*t*

growth
  in children, 250–251
  ICS and, 184

H

H1N1 virus, 219, 224, 226*t*
Handihaler, 155
Harlem, asthma in, 7
Helicobacter pylori, 26
HEPA. *See* high-efficiency particulate air
hepatitis, 179
herbal remedies, for asthma, 194–197
HFA. *See* hydrofluoroalkane
high-efficiency particulate air (HEPA),
    229–231
hormone, 171
hydrofluoroalkane (HFA)
  cleaning of, 147, 148*t*
  criteria of, 188
  dosing of, 149
  experts' view of, 148*t*
  facts about, 146*t*
  generic, 148*t*
  medicine in, 144–145
  priming of, 146*t*
  spray of, 147
hygiene hypothesis, 25
  epidemiology of, 26
hyperreactivity, 30, 31*t*
hypercarbic pattern, 123
hyperinflation, 57
hypertension, 201
hypoxemic pattern, 123

I

ICS. *See* inhaled corticosteroids
IgE. *See* immunoglobulin E
immune system, causing asthma, 13
ImmunoCAP blood test, 111–112
immunoglobulin, 115
immunoglobulin E (IgE), 115
  blockers, 192
  discovery of, 189
  effects of, at cellular level, 191
  levels of, 111
    measurement of, 191
immunologist, 86
immunomodulator, 130*t*
immunotherapy, for allergies, 113–114
in vitro, 111
in vivo, 112
indoor allergen, 264
indoor environment, 17*f*
  Clearing the Air: Asthma and Indoor Air, 21

inflammation
  chronic, 92, 173
  contemporary view of, 30*t*
  definition of, 28
  recognition of, 31
influenza
  asthma and, 219–227
  definition of, 219
  facts about, 220*t*
  prevention of, 222
  seasonal, 221, 223*t*
  seasonal vaccine for, comparison of, 225*t*
  strains of, 224
  vaccine against, 222–223, 223*t*
    doctors checking you before, 227
inhaled corticosteroids (ICS)
  in asthma, 173*t*
  classification of, 130*t*
  efficacy of, 172
  facts about, 129*t*
  generic/trade names of, 131*t*
  growth and, 184
  LABA combined with, 132*t*
  quality from, 175
  safety of, 182–183
  side effects of, 183*t*
inhaled cromolyn, 130*t*
inhaler. *See also* dry-powder inhaler;
    metered-dose inhaler
  benefits of, 141
  breathing for, 156
  delivery via, 133*t*
  HFA, 146–147
  nebulizer v., 169–171
  types of, 141
  uses of, 133*t*
  Using Inhaled Devices, 156
inspiratory, 38
  action, 51
International Study of Asthma and Allergies
    in Childhood (ISAAC), 6
internist, 106
internship, 103
ipratropium (Atrovent), 130*t*
ISAAC. *See* International Study of Asthma
    and Allergies in Childhood

J

jogging, cough after, 41–42

L

LABA. *See* long-acting β₂ agonists
LAIV. *See* live, attenuated influenza vaccine
laryngeal dysfunction, 44*t*

larynx, 41, 125
leptin, role of, 204
leukotriene, 213
leukotriene modifiers, 130*t*
   control with, 134
   exercise and, 213–214
   generic/trade names for, 131*t*
   uses of, 134
leukotriene receptor antagonist (LTRA), 134
levalbuterol (Xopenex), 129*t*–131*t*, 132,
     133*t*, 134
live, attenuated influenza vaccine (LAIV),
     224–225
long-acting β₂ agonists (LABA), 130*t*
   examples of, 189
   generic/trade names of, 132*t*
   ICS combined with, 132*t*
   inhaler delivery of, 133*t*
loose bowels, 179
LTRA. *See* leukotriene receptor antagonist
lungs
   ailments of, 47
   anatomy of, 10*f*, 11
   after birth, 12
   diseases of, 44, 44*t*
   NHLBI, 189
   symptoms of, 43
   volume of, 58*t*
   workings of, 9, 10*f*

M

magnetic resonance imaging (MRI), 57
Martinez, Dr. Fernando, 204–205
Maternal Vitamin D Supplementation to
     Prevent Childhood Asthma
     (VDAART), 14
Maxair (pirbuterol), 129*t*–131*t*, 132–134,
     133*t*, 138
MDI. *See* metered-dose inhaler
mediators, 173
medical schools, 103
medications. *See also* asthma medications
   for COPD, 47
   generic names of, 131*t*–132*t*, 134*t*
   in HFA, 144–145
   inhaler delivery of, 133*t*
   liquid form of, 171
   for nebulizer, 168
     inhaler v., 169–171
   safe, 84*t*
   stopping of, 93
   trade names of, 131*t*–132*t*, 134*t*
Medrol (methylprednisolone), 178

metered-dose inhaler (MDI), 99, 119
   actuation of, 163
   CFCs in, 143–144
   common errors in, 159*t*
   concepts of, 157
   empty, 161–162
   reformulated albuterol, 144
   rinsing mouth after, 159–163, 159*t*
   safety of, 182–183
   shaking of, 161
   storage of, 156
   use of, 141
     correct, 155–159
     technique for, 158
   VHC with, 164–165
methacholine challenge, 62–63
methylprednisolone (Medrol), 178
methylxanthines, 130*t*
Meticorten (prednisone)
   side effects of, 180
   use of, 178
milk
   asthma and, 249*t*, 250
   side effects of, 250
mineral supplements, for asthma, 197–202
monometasone (Asmanex), 130*t*, 131*t*,
     133*t*, 151–152
montelukast (Singulair), 134*t*
Montreal Protocol, 141–144
morbidity, 68
mortality, 68
MRI. *See* magnetic resonance imaging
mucus
   definition of, 2
   hypersecretion of, 35*t*
myths, about asthma, 232*t*

N

NAEPP. *See* National Asthma Education
     and Prevention Program
National Asthma Education and Prevention
     Program (NAEPP), 68
   classification by, 71
   contemporary approaches of, 188
   measurements for, 58*t*, 59
   for older children/adults, 101
National Center for Complementary and
     Alternative Medicine (NCCAM),
     195–196
National Heart, Lung, and Blood Institute
     (NHLBI), 189
NCCAM. *See* National Center for Comple-
     mentary and Alternative Medicine

nebulizer
    characteristics of, 166
    in emergency room, 119
    guidelines for, 167
    mechanics of, 167
    medications used in, 168
        inhaler v., 169–171
    patient experience of, 169
    type of, 97
nedocromil sodium (Tilade MDI), 130*t*
New York City, air quality in, 233
NHLBI. *See* National Heart, Lung,
        and Blood Institute
Nighttime reflux, 52
nocturnal awakenings, 35*t*,
        139–140
nocturnal symptoms, 34
nonelectrostatic chambers, 164
non-steroidal anti-inflammatory drugs
        (NSAIDs)
    causing attacks, 83
    definition of, 82
NSAIDs. *See* non-steroidal
        anti-inflammatory drugs
nutrition, 199–202
    in pregnancy, 200

O

obesity
    asthma and, 202–207
    definition of, 202
    determination of, 206–207
    medical risks with, 205–206
    and OSAS, 49
obstructive dysfunction, characteristics
        of, 45–46
occupational asthma, 85
    types of, 87
occupational exposures, 50*t*
Olympic winter sports athletes, 81
omalizumab (Xolair), 130*t*, 138, 189, 191,
        192*t*, 243
open-mouth technique, 156
oral, 78
OSAS. *See* obesity and obstructive sleep
        apnea syndrome
osteopath, 103
osteopathy, 105
osteoporosis
    GIO, 181
    Vitamin D and, 201*t*
outdoor environment, 17*f*
oxygen (O$_2$)

in breathing, 11–12
    functions of, 64
    insufficient, 123
    loss of, 101–102
    supplemental, 119
ozone, 142, 215

P

pandemic, 219
Pari Vortex, 164
pathologic, 174
patient education, in asthma action plan,
        87–88
peak expiratory flow (PEF)
    devices for, 61
    in emergency room, 120
    importance of, 60–61
    performance of, 59
    red-zone, 118
    as subtest, 58
peak-flow meter, 61
peak-flow monitoring, 61–62
pediatrician, 106
Pediatrics, 202
PEF. *See* peak expiratory flow
percussion, 55
Performist (formoterol solution), 132*t*
pets
    allergies to, 263–265
    in school, 265
PFTs. *See* pulmonary function tests
pharmacotherapy, 113
physical education, 257
physical examination, for asthma, 55
physician
    qualifications of, 104*t*
    types of, 103
PIE. *See* pulmonary infiltrates with
        eosinophilia
pirbuterol (Maxair), 129*t*–131*t*, 132,
        133*t*
plural bronchi, 9
postnasal drip, 43
pranayama yoga, 216
prednisone (Meticorten)
    side effects of, 180
    use of, 178
pregnancy
    asthma and, 236, 238
    asthma medications during, 240–243
        classification of, 241*t*
    asthma prevention during, 238–240, 238*t*
    asthma specialist during, 236–238

pregnancy (*continued*)
  cigarette smoking during, 239
  nutrition in, 200
  outcome of, 237
premenstrual asthma, 197
prevalence
  of asthma, 6–7, 6*t*
  definition of, 25
prevention
  of asthma, 20–25
    prenatal, 238–240
  NAEPP, 58*t*, 59, 68, 71, 101, 188
primary care pediatrician, 253–255
ProAir (albuterol sulfate), 133*t*, 138, 144,
    146–147, 148*t*
Professional Association of Diving
    Instructors, 218
propellant. *See* hydrofluoroalkane
Proventil (albuterol sulfate), 131*t*, 133*t*,
    138–139, 144, 146–147, 148*t*
psychological disease, asthma as,
    231–233
puberty, 205
Pulmicort (budesonide), 131*t*
pulmonary embolus, 48
pulmonary function lab, 63
pulmonary function tests (FEV), 69, 70*t*
  as subtest, 57–58
pulmonary function tests (PFTs)
  history of, 57
  uses of, 55–57
pulmonary infiltrates with eosinophilia
    (PIE), 49
pulmonary symptoms, 54
pulmonologist, 65
pulse oximeter, 102

Q

quick-relief asthma medications, 129
  choice of, 132
  names of, 131*t*
  in night, 140
quiescent asthma, 29*t*
Qvar (beclomethasone), 131*t*, 133*t*,
    144

R

RadioAllergo-Sorbent Test (RAST),
    111
radiographic testing, 56*t*
RADS, 87
RAST. *See* RadioAllergo-Sorbent Test
Reclast (zoledronic acid), 182
Recommended Dietary Allowances, 199

ReliOn (albuterol sulfate), 131*t*, 133*t*, 134,
    148–149
remission, 29
residency, 103
respiration, 10*f*
  cycle of, 51
  definition of, 64
respiratory failure
  causes of, 124
  death from, 124
  definition of, 64, 123
respiratory rate, 12
respiratory system
  functions of, 64
  viral infections in, 50*t*
retraction, 118
rhinitis, 49, 50*t*, 134
rigid bronchoscopy, 66
rinsing mouth, after MDI use, 159–163
risk factors
  for asthma, 122–123, 122*t*
  of asthma medications, during
      pregnancy, 241*t*
  for cancer, 201*t*
  for obesity, 205–206

S

SABA. *See* short-acting β₂ bronchodilator
safety
  of asthma medications, during
      pregnancy, 240–243
  of ICS, 182–183
  of MDI, 182–183
  of steroids, 177–178
salmeterol (Serevent), 130*t*, 132*t*–133*t*,
    151
school staff, 257–259
school-age children
  pets for, 265
  wheezing in, 247–248
scuba diving, asthma and, 217–219
secondhand smoke, 21, 262–263
self-monitoring, of asthma, 61
sensitization, 111
Serevent (salmeterol), 130*t*, 132*t*–133*t*, 151
short-acting β₂ bronchodilator (SABA), 71
  classification of, 128, 130*t*
  facts about, 129*t*
  generic/trade names of, 134
  inhaler delivery of, 133*t*
shortness of breath, 44*t*
side effects
  from asthma treatment, 179–185
  of corticosteroids, 179–185

of ICS, 183*t*
of milk, 250
of prednisone, 180
Singulair (montelukast), 134*t*, 138
sinuses, anatomy of, 42
sinusitis, 49–50
sleep, asthma and, 139–140
smoking. *See* cigarette smoking
spacers, 165, 165*t*
Spiriva (tiotropium), 130*t*, 150
spirometry, 46, 55
    components of, 58*t*
    importance of, 57–58
    performance of, 59
sports
    asthma and, 209–216
    Olympic winter, athletes, 81
    symptoms after, 41–42
steroids. *See also* corticosteroids; inhaled
        corticosteroids
    anabolic, 176
    dangers of, 175–179
    endogenous, 176
    patient experience with,
        178–179
    safety of, 177–178
    types of, 178
    use guidelines for, 177
stethoscope, 38
Still, Andrew Taylor, 105
stomach, acid in, 52
Strachan, David, 25
sulfite additives, sensitivity to, 50*t*
supplements
    for asthma, 197–202
    VDAART, 14
sustained release theophylline
        (Theocron), 130*t*
swimming, 212
Symbicort (budesonide-formoterol),
        132*t*–133*t*, 162

T

Theochron (sustained release theophylline),
        131*t*
therapeutic use exemption (TUE), 80
Tilade MDI (nedocromil sodium), 133*t*
tiotropium (Spiriva), 130*t*, 150
Title VI of the Clean Air Act, 143
tobacco smoke, 50*t*
    ETS, 21–22
    secondhand, 21, 262–263
tools, for asthma diagnosis, 56*t*
trachea, 9

trade names
    FDA approval of, 138
    generic names v., 137–139
    of medications, 131*t*–132*t*, 134*t*
triamcinolone (Azmacort), 130*t*–131*t*, 133*t*
trigger
    definition of, 19
    emotional response as, 232–233
    exercise as, 42, 210
    types of, 96–97
tuberculosis, 179
TUE. *See* therapeutic use exemption
Twisthaler, 154–155

U

United States
    Anti-Doping Agency, 80
    asthma in, 4*t*
    National Academy of Sciences' National
        Research Council, 199
urticaria, 115

V

vaccine
    asthma and, 225
    definition of, 219
    against influenza, 222–223
        doctors checking you before, 227
    seasonal, 225
valved holding chamber (VHC),
        163–166
    benefits of, 165
    MDI with, 164–165
    patient experience of, 166
VCD. *See* vocal cord dysfunction
VDAART. *See* Maternal Vitamin
        D Supplementation to Prevent
        Childhood Asthma
ventilator, uses of, 65
Ventolin (albuterol sulfate), 131*t*, 133*t*, 134,
        138, 144–145, 146–149
    empty, 161–162
VHC. *See* valved holding chamber
viral, 77
virus
    asthmagenic, 14
    definition of, 219
    H1N1, 219, 224, 226*t*
    respiratory infections from, 50*t*
vitamins
    for asthma, 197–202
    categories of, 199
    for children, 250
    D, 200–201, 201*t*

vitamins (*continued*)
  deficiencies of, 199
  VDAART, 14
vocal cord dysfunction (VCD)
  diagnosis of, 51–52
  discovery of, 50
  symptoms of, 44, 51
  wheezing and, 41
vocal cords, 51
Vortex, 164

W

water retention, 180
wheeze, 35*t*
  in babies, 251*t*
  beta-blocker-induced, 44*t*, 50
  causes of, 40, 40*t*, 248
  COPD and, 40, 40*t*
  creation of, 38

definition of, 2, 37
detection of, 39
example of, 38–39
in school-age children, 247–248
VCD and, 41
work-related asthma, 86

X

Xolair (omalizumab), 138, 192*t*
Xopenex (levalbuterol), 129*t*–131*t*,
  132–134, 133*t*

Z

zafirlukast (Accolate), 134*t*
zileuton (Zyflo), 130–131, 134*t*
Zoledroniczileuton (Zyflo), 130–131,
  134*t*
zoledronic acid (Reclast), 182
Zyflo (zileuton), 130–131, 134*t*